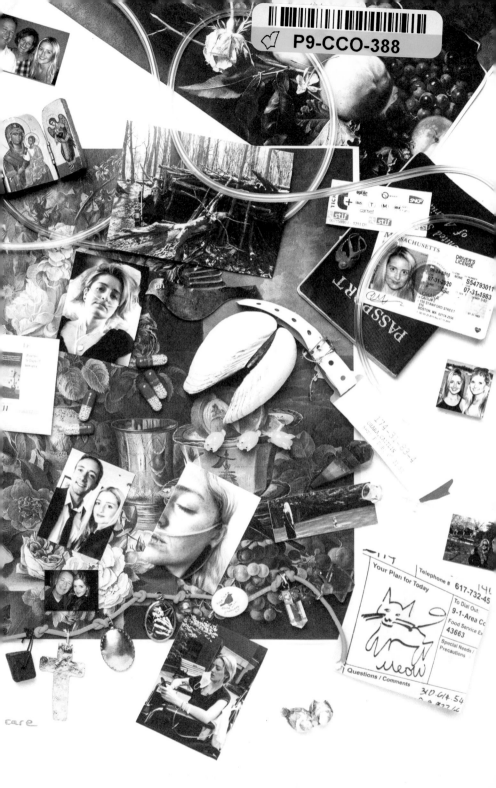

"This is a book about life, including death. For showing us how to hold both, we owe Maryanne and Caitlin a magnificent debt of gratitude. Here is love in ink, and you will feel it. That's not to say that their story is easy to behold—you will cry—but that's key to the book's great achievement: within a connection like theirs, *everything* has a home. Despair, hope, fear, beauty, decay, out of this world, in this world. It turns out that death poses no threat to love. Read this book to help you know that in your bones."

—B. J. Miller, author of *A Beginner's Guide to the End*

"To the stalwart scientists and physicians who go to battle in service of the seriously sick, who peer into microscopes and imagine the unseeable deep within to discover cures, I urge you to pick up your heads and look through the lens of Maryanne O'Hara's *Little Matches* to fully understand your power, to know what is at stake in your pursuits to transform hope to joy, tears to laughter, and to feel the weight of what happens if we fail."

—Patrick R. Connelly, PhD, Senior Vertex Fellow, Vertex Pharmaceuticals

"Maryanne O'Hara has written an extraordinary book, beautiful, heartbreaking, and so full of life on every page that I was reminded that loving deeply is full of risk and the only way to live. This is the most meaningful book I've read in a very long time."

—Jane Bernstein, author of *The Face Tells the Secret* and *Rachel in the World*

LITTLE MATCHES

LITTLE
MATCHES

A Memoir of Grief and Light

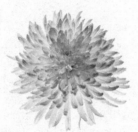

MARYANNE O'HARA

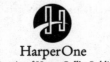

HarperOne
An Imprint of HarperCollinsPublishers

HarperCollins books may be purchased for educational, business, or sales promotional use. For information, please email the Special Markets Department at SPsales@harpercollins.com.

FIRST EDITION

Flower art by Yulia Mladich/Shutterstock, Inc.
Endpapers photograph by Winky Lewis

Library of Congress Cataloging-in-Publication Data is available upon request.

ISBN 978-0-06-302776-3

21 22 23 24 25 LSC 10 9 8 7 6 5 4 3 2 1

For "Nick and Dad"
for Andrew and Jess and Katie
and for every kind stranger

CONTENTS

PREFACE

Little Matches is a book about losing my beloved only child and my search for answers to the hard questions. *Where is she? Is she? Is there more to life than this life? Does consciousness survive death? Does my existence have any real purpose? Does anyone's?*

It's also an exploration of the growth I experienced as parent and friend to a gift of a human being.

And it's a meditation on universal truths about loving and losing and needing human connection.

Caitlin was born with a genetic, progressive disease—in her case, cystic fibrosis (CF)—and like many children who live with serious illness, she was wiser than her years. As she grew sicker, and particularly as she grew into an adult, she became a kind of sage for those around her. She often joked that if she hadn't had CF, she might have been a shallow sort of person, which was her modest way of pointing out that she didn't think she was particularly special, it was just that having to face your mortality makes you look at life, and the world, with a much broader and deeper perspective.

She was right. People who face trauma, illness, or severe loss often find themselves transformed, and come to question or better understand what life is "really for."

During her long wait for a lung transplant, I used a blog, *9Lives Notes.com*, to keep loved ones abreast of news. After her passing, I kept it alive and every time I posted something—an insight of my own, or some of Caitlin's old-soul wisdom—I would receive what I called the "you don't know me letters." *You don't know me but*, they would begin, and go on to say how helpful it was to read honest, unsentimental reflections on suffering and loss, and on the mysteries that connect us as human beings who find ourselves alive, with questions, on a wild and nurturing planet.

People also found inspiration in my accounts of our strong mother-daughter bond, in how Caitlin's wise words and ways became sources of insight and hope, even after her passing. These readers asked for more stories. They urged me to turn the blog into a book.

Even though writing the blog posts had been my salvation, at first I was too catatonic with grief to even think of tackling a book. But nine months after her passing, I realized I was adrift, that I no longer had any kind of rudder. If my writing about Caitlin was going to serve a purpose, then I wanted to do it.

I had to decide how to distill the material of our story into one that could inspire readers to contemplate for themselves what might really matter at the end of our temporary, beautiful lives. Here is what I came up with. I start with a chapter called "Knowing," wherein I put myself and my reader right inside the worst of it: the stunning, sudden loss of Caitlin. I call this one-chapter section Book One: "In Between." I keep the reader close as I grope my way through the dark and take refuge in old journals, those proofs of days otherwise forgotten, to return to her beginnings, which is Book Two: "Life," made up of chapters 2 through 12.

Here I follow a mostly chronological order, moving us through time by way of meditations that include glimpses of the web that was our daily human life—snippets of text messages, emails, journal entries, lists, even drawings—with the section ending where the book began. In Book Three: "Afterlife," which includes chapters 13 through 17, I document the wasteland I traveled through for the first two years after Caitlin's passing, at which point something in me told me it was time to find a bigger purpose. Finally, in the afterword, I put in some pieces written by or about Caitlin that may be of interest. These are followed by a list of books and resources for those who would like more information on the various topics that I discuss in the book.

In real time, I looked for revelation. I became every human who has ever looked for answers to big life questions inside books and science and in the natural world and inside personal relationships. As the narrator of my own story I moved back and forth through time, much like memory works, and came to focus on a few ideas: that purpose in life is necessary, and probably a prerequisite to joy and contentment; that by acknowledging the inevitability of our mortality, we can actually better enjoy the time we are alive; that we are all connected; and that we all have work to do.

I am not the first person to have lost what was most important to me. Humans lose every day, and lose hard: children, beloveds, sacred homelands, freedoms. *Little Matches* is for anyone who loses and asks, *Now what?*

When Caitlin was clinging to life during her final days, she called us to her bedside. She was serious, fierce. "Listen, she said, "I need ferocious positivity from everyone."

Ferocious positivity isn't a meme or a passed-around quote. Ferocious positivity is here, in her last posted words:

My thoughts these days aren't the skate-on-top kind of normal life thoughts. They're up and down and trippy and depressive—and we have a lot of laughs. And lots of crying. And weird creative urges. I just want to say thank you for listening to what sometimes must be very emotionally over-the-top sounding writing. And to reassure you I don't take myself too seriously. I do take life seriously though, I'll be honest . . . because it's a seriously wild business.

Life *is* a seriously wild business. And it's all ours, for a little while.

Someone recently referred to *Little Matches* as a "healing garden of words." The metaphor took me by surprise. The speaker had just met me, and he did not know that Caitlin had spent the last two years of her life trying to save a world-renowned hospital healing garden. He did not know that since her passing, I had been trying to think of how I could create a kind of physical, real-life "portable healing garden," a place where people might find whatever comfort and inspiration they needed. I wasn't even sure what a physical, real-life portable healing garden would look like. Now I think it might look like *Little Matches*.

Book One

In Between

*In the middle of our life's journey, I
found myself in a dark wood.*

—DANTE

1

KNOWING

It's as horrible as I knew it would be. It is silent, internal hysteria, and it is unbearable.

People say, "I can't imagine," and I think, *Really? You can't imagine?*

Maybe having healthy children protects you from letting your mind go to the darkest places.

One friend says, "I'm so sorry. I don't know how you can close your eyes at night."

Here's how I do it: I close my eyes. I ask the universe to give me an hour of unconsciousness. Somehow it works.

I'm learning to talk to the universe.

I think, *I can bear it if I know I will see her again.*

I nonstop devour the kinds of books she and I sometimes liked to read and discuss. I call them "soul" books: *We Don't Die; Many Lives, Many Masters; The Light Between Us.* These particular books are intelligently written, credible, and they provide some comfort in the moment. *Yes,* they say, *we birth into this life knowing, at a soul level, our life's plan. Yes, there is more to life than this life.*

When I close them, I'm a frantic human mother again, sick with doubt and grief.

❦

We are all so present in these two worlds we live in—the old natural world of relationships, of day-to-day existence, combined now with our digital selves, our presence in ten thousand photographs and videos—that the abrupt absence of any one of us, overnight, seems exponentially impossible.

We say what humans have always said, *I can't believe I will never see her again.* Yet there she is, talking from the small screen in my palm. There she is, *existing.* Disbelief compounded.

The brain gifts us with that disbelief. At the instant of comprehension, it shuts down, protecting us, I suppose, by feeding us small bits of reality at a time.

The only thing that makes me feel better, makes me feel connected to her, is writing on *9LivesNotes.com*, the website I set up just before she was formally listed, on April 24, 2014, for a double lung transplant, the end-of-the-line fix for people with severe cystic fibrosis. We had heard of people who had had to wait up to a year— sometimes even longer—but the transplant team stressed that the call really could come at any time.

We trusted that it would.

Lung transplantation is a risky surgery, and there are no guarantees, but we knew so many success stories, people who had skidded right up to the edge of death yet come out the other side. They skied and hiked and visited China and went to work each day. Their stories kept us realistically optimistic.

Caitlin kept us optimistic, too. As she grew into adulthood, she became as medically knowledgeable as any doctor. She took meticulous, disciplined care of herself and had survived decades of health scares. From babyhood, her tongue-in-cheek nickname had been Kitten Caitlin. She had nine lives. Or so we thought. What happened to her should not have happened to anyone, and I need to make some kind of sense of it.

Maybe the example of her life is supposed to be some kind of help to others. Judging from the abundance of correspondence that I am receiving, from strangers who have only heard about her and are grateful for her wisdom, her example, that is a reasonable assumption. The fact of her existence certainly bettered my own.

Or maybe nothing means anything. I'm trying to figure it all out.

On Caitlin's first day on life support, when she was still conscious and able to speak, her ICU nurse mentioned having been to Mass the day before.

CAITLIN: *Do you believe in God?*
NURSE: *I do.*
CAITLIN: *Why?*
NURSE: *Why not?*

I wish I had the ability to remember, in detail, all that Caitlin said, but basically she talked about how she believed in something greater but thought that the various religions hadn't gotten it right.

Now I think: *Now she knows.* All the stuff we talked about is no longer theoretical for one of us.

It is disorienting to be home, in this house I longed for while we were banished to Pittsburgh for two years. Pittsburgh, for a bunch of reasons, being the only medical center that would transplant her. That additional injustice.

It's Christmastime and the house is full of people. They float around the edges of my consciousness. My sister has multiplied. She is everywhere, doing, helping. I move through people's kindnesses like a ghost, drifting up to my second floor. From my chair I can look up from my soul books and out over the frozen river, comforted by the fact that loved ones are down there without actually having to interact with anyone.

Food is dust.

I have lost fifteen pounds.

Nick comes in and out. I am careful and kind with him. He has lost his daughter, too.

It was all so close.

❦

As I stumble inside this world Caitlin grew up in, I discover something: when you lose a child, all the separate ages they ever were become newly present. My daughter is no longer just thirty-three but all of the ages she ever was.

She is three and I am driving her to preschool when I hear her squeaky voice from the back seat: "Maybe I'll make some friends."

I walk into the kitchen and she's there with her hands planted on her hips, face wet with exasperated tears, scolding me in a scene we laughed about for years. "Don't you *know?* Don't you *know* you're not supposed to shout at a little girl like me?"

In the airport, I am laden with bags and need to let go of her hand. "Now stay right here," I say as she cackles and takes off, shouting, *"I'm a baaaad girl!"*

The school years are an arc of images: a miniature adult in first grade, consoling a scared, sobbing friend. In high school, telling me about a new girl named Jess who is "funny and smart and nice" and how there is "just something about Jess. I feel like I have to protect her."

Caitlin was innately kind in a way I was not when I was young. I always marveled at that. Where did that goodness come from? And that fire that was there from the beginning?

The Boston Globe is running a front-page feature obituary, the *Boston Herald* and *MetroWest Daily News* publishing prominent pieces as well. At one point a reporter and photographer interview Caitlin's boyfriend and me and set us up for a photograph—Caitlin's little dog on my lap, grieving Andrew by my side.

I shrink from the clichéd tableau.

A week ago, Caitlin was this season's holiday miracle. Now she is its tragedy.

Nick is not with us because he is the brave one, in town, facing all the decisions the funeral director is pressing on us to make and that my own brain recoils from.

Andrew squeezes my hand and I squeeze his back, grateful for him and for Nick, and for all the people, loved ones, and strangers alike who are shouldering a share of this hideous grief.

I am back to my own beginnings, that awakening to my own existence, when I had little to think about but what is this world, why is this world?

The soul books get me remembering odd happenings from my earliest days.

Being very young and wondering why people were afraid of pain because I knew that all you had to do in dire circumstances was "jump out of your body."

Floating fevered in my childhood bed, adult faces looming close, my hands like those two balloons Pink Floyd sang about. That vague, almost grasping of *something*.

Sitting in my third-grade classroom filled with a sudden, urgent sense that I had made a mistake with this life, that I needed to start over, that I *could*.

And as a young adult, hospitalized after minor surgery, Nick beside me, we discovered that I "knew" what he was thinking, and vice versa. It sounds weird, but it really happened. We made a game of it, but it only lasted as long as that brief, inpatient night in the hospital.

Have most people had these kinds of experiences? Caitlin's final weeks in the hospital were marked by striking synchronicities, and when I share them, the unlikeliest, most commonsense people begin telling me stories. The dying woman who said, "You're going to think I'm crazy but my sister's here." The cat that dropped dead, literally, during a mother's funeral and the random stranger who told the daughter, years later, "Your mother's fine; the cat's with her." The voice that said, "Go outside," at the time of a father's passing and outside was a radiant sunset and "the sense of his presence ten feet away and to my left."

There are so many such stories of people's last hours. Their observations, their words. The way Steve Jobs looked past his loved ones and said, *Oh wow. Oh wow. Oh wow.*

I huddle on the cold stone steps at the end of our lawn, looking out over the frozen river. Wintry gusts skitter leaf debris across the surface of the ice. Under it, the moving water makes sounds from science fiction—reverberating warps and booms. The ice is alive, with cracks that branch like trees and broccoli and the bronchi of human lungs.

Fractals, the natural world astonishing us with its mathematical marvels. Patterns that suggest design, intent, meaning.

There is more to life than me, than us.

That thought has helped me from my earliest days.

We lived through the dawn of the digital age. AOL, AIM, gmail, gchats, iPhone iMessages. So much material. Conversations that would normally have been spoken and lost forever exist in long, scrolling pages. It's all here.

We have not yet announced a service, but I have set myself the task of choosing images and words for the book-like program I need to assemble and for the tribute film that I have asked my artist brother to create. I have immersed myself in Caitlin's phone, my phone, our computers, old family videotapes, and all my years of journals, those records of days that might otherwise have been forgotten.

I dip into and out of the past and the past becomes the present and I am living inside my present-past and it is the only comfort.

I have been sending Caitlin text messages.

When she was unconscious in the ICU, I would write, *I miss you, bud. So many things I go to tell you, just silly things, like Pup. Puppetypuppup! I'm sending these now for us to laugh at later.*

Her name was always at the top of my iMessages list. Now I have to scroll down, down, down to find her.

MARYANNE: Where are you?

I love you.

I love you.

I am in pain.

I love you.

Over forever.

I love you.

So much.

I miss you.

Where are you? Fuck this.

❧

Somewhere online, I see a meme, attributed to the artist Barbara Kruger, that makes sense to me: Belief + Doubt = Sanity.

I wonder if it is possible to mix up that equation. To add doubt to sanity and arrive at belief.

That comforting stack of soul books—if I accept their premise that I chose this life, planned this course to challenge myself, well, if that's all true, then everything that has happened can make some kind of sense.

Because for many years, I have felt that things that were happening seemed part of some predetermined script. There has been so much *knowing*.

Before the cystic fibrosis diagnosis, Caitlin had been hospitalized with pneumonia, treated, and discharged. All was now "well," but as I was climbing the stairs to unpack her suitcase, I paused on the top tread. Something in me just *knew*. It wasn't over.

Most CF patients culture *pseudomonas*, a bacterium that causes steady, ongoing lung damage. But an outbreak of a particularly vicious, virulent bacterium—*Burkholderia cepacia*—at Cleveland Clinic in the late 1980s caused rapid deterioration and death in many CF patients. When I panicked, Caitlin's pulmonologist told me not to worry. Ohio was far from Boston, and yes, cepacia was scary, and highly resistant to drugs, but only 3 percent of CF patients ever cultured it. Still, I knew in my gut that we were going to have to deal with it, and years later, despite all of my over-the-top precautions, we did.

From babyhood until school days, Caitlin grew up with a girl, Hillary, born just one week after her own birth. Hillary's mother, a former teacher, was our neighbor and a perfect child-minder. When the girls were one, we moved out of our rented place to a home we bought a few towns away. Many years later, Caitlin's lifelong chest physical therapist, who treated her at our house every school day morning, took on another CF patient. One day she talked about the little girl's apartment, and how the girl's mom, a single mother, worked so hard to make it nice. She began to describe it, and I said, "Wait a minute." And yes, it was the very same apartment where we lived the first year of Caitlin's life.

In December 2007, Hillary, recently married, with a master's in public health from Yale and a bright new career in Texas, became suddenly ill with acute leukemia. She died on December 21, nine years, nearly to the minute, before Caitlin.

I don't know that any of that means anything. It doesn't help my sanity equation.

For most of my adult life, I had a major, overarching identity—mother/caregiver to a sick child. For the past three years, waiting for transplant, every day was consumed by that role. I couldn't have filled it as well as I did without Nick and Andrew, but their support meant I was able to be *the one*.

Now what am I for?

Am I supposed to do something with the experience? Share Caitlin's wise, written reflections of the past few years, when being dependent on supplemental oxygen meant that writing was easier than speaking? Share the uncanny yet comforting synchronicities that have marked our days?

I am ruminating on all this when a young friend from Pittsburgh sends me a note:

I remember so clearly meeting Caitlin for the first time. We had met you and Nick just a bit before and it was such a nice surprise to step into the elevator of 151 and see you and Caitlin. She turned her head, slowly removed her sunglasses and looked up and smiled and introduced herself. I had never seen someone make a wheelchair look glamorous, but she did. When we got off the elevator I remember saying to my husband, "She's just so beautiful, so so beautiful." I was slightly in awe of the way she glowed.

You once asked me if we could hear you from our condo below you—I think I said something about the vacuum cleaner. But the other thing we could hear was the oxygen tanks moving around. You could hear them clink on the floor. I didn't know what it was until I heard it in the garage. After realizing what it was,

I developed a habit of praying for Caitlin every time I heard the clink. I never told her that I prayed for her, or how often I thought of you all upstairs, I didn't want her to think that I pitied her, or for her to feel self-conscious or that I was invading her privacy. Now, I find that slightly stupid of me, I didn't have to tell her the way I was reminded to pray for her, but why wouldn't you tell someone that you care? Why not risk feeling awkward or silly for the sake of someone else?

Why not indeed? Her words remind me of a book I recently read, by a hospice chaplain who said something to the effect of *You need to know this: everyone is broken.*

I have always resisted writing about my personal life, but I suspect that I am supposed to document this time. Let people know that none of us is alone with our broken bits.

I think, too, of the message I ignored a few years back.

You're supposed to help people into the next life.

⸎

From: Caitlin
To: A friend with CF who'd had a successful lung transplant
Date: July 25, 2014
Subject: Other things

I am reading Primo Levi's *Periodic Table* right now, and every night it's like a tonic—I only read one chapter / one element. Do you know it? I share a birthday with him, and maybe I know too much about astrology and am unfairly influenced, but I can't help but feel an incredible kinship to and relation to his writing. I have read his other memoirs of being in Auschwitz. They are hard to read yes, but more I feel like a window into a study of humanity that most of us will luckily never see . . . but should at least read about.

I've done a lot of soul searching (cheesy term but true) the past year, and I've read a few things that have been helpful. One thing I re-read was Emerson's "Self Reliance," which I only remembered from college and high school, but it's cathartic to just read the philosophies that are so aligned with what I feel like I know I can trust fully and have full faith in—that is—myself, my intuition. And also *Gilead* by Marilynne Robinson. I am always fascinated by people who are really intelligent and intellectual and yet still very Christian—or return to religion after a lifetime of academia (that is not me, but it interests me how those two opposing sides manage to come together). Also this book of Tolstoy's, *A Confession*. It's really small and he wrote it at the end of his life when he was practically suicidal because he was driven so insane by his inability to have faith, and his in-vain attempts to arrive at it logically. I've re-read that many times over the years (it has a good conclusion) and what you said about surrendering—I completely agree that the moments when I have felt most free, most OK with what is happening, and least anxious, have been those moments where I am able to let go and surrender.

Interestingly, those moments seem to work in tandem with my faith in myself. I know I can trust myself to get through something, to hold on, and ultimately I can just let go of the rest. So I guess since we have no idea where we come from, and where that strength comes from . . . that true belief in yourself and your intent to be a good person is sort of divine in itself, no more or less divine than believing in something someone else told you to believe in. I have always believed in goodness and I know a lot of people say that, but it does feel undeniably essential, and I don't question it. As humans we somehow know that we should aim to be good, and where does that come from? If I can follow the fact that I can trust in the importance of goodness, then I can maybe trust that goodness will come of goodness . . . if that makes sense. Kind of like karma points. I have never felt like "why did this happen to me" as I am sure you haven't either. It isn't even because of some virtue that I feel that way, it just has never occurred to me to be "pissed off" about my lot in life, or to think that there was some unjust reasoning behind it. Instead I honestly feel lucky sometimes that I have gotten to feel and experience things that others have to struggle longer and harder to learn.

Book Two

Life

It's part of why the idea of souls makes sense to me. This place is just like a ropes course for souls. A learning center. It never changes and the collective body of humans can never sustain their progress too too much or else there is not enough to challenge the souls. Imagine all the people living life in peace—John Lennon ✄—well that wouldn't really work if you believe we need to be challenged to grow.

—CAITLIN O'HARA

2

RELUCTANT MOTHER

11/1/2008

MARYANNE: bay scallop ceviche. shrimp toasts.
CAITLIN: stop im so hungry
MARYANNE: did you look at our party pictures
CAITLIN: yeah they are good
MARYANNE: how about daddy, in the role of angel !!?? haha
CAITLIN: daddy looks so funny
hahah it was funny
MARYANNE: eyes cast heavenward, playing the harp
CAITLIN: ha
did you see mine
MARYANNE: yes, i saw them. you looked so beautiful
i can't believe how beautiful you are sometimes
it's like when you were a baby and i used to stare at your perfect
little face

Nick and I met by accident. Or by fate, depending on your point of view. I was twenty years old, spending my college summers in Ireland and randomly visited his hometown. He was there one night more than planned because his car had broken down as he'd been about to head back to London, where he was living. We met, clicked, and dated each summer for a couple of years.

Nick: he's an extrovert with a sense of humor and Irish accent that lets him get away with a lot, but he's also one of the most honorable and kind-hearted people I know. A friend recently described him as "respectfully inappropriate." He comes across as easygoing but he is also ambitious and driven and clever and artistic and Ireland in the 1980s was way too small for him. He saw all of America as one big, beckoning Statue of Liberty, and the year I graduated from college, he came for a visit and never went back. He had an idea for a design and construction business that would execute his particular vision of "artistry in masonry." We married early and, one month after the ceremony, found ourselves unexpectedly expecting.

I had never especially wanted kids and certainly hadn't planned on one now, but Nick, who'd grown up among large Irish families, took the news in stride.

We didn't anticipate any health problems. The only thing I worried about, never having felt maternal, was that I would not feel anything for the baby.

Don't worry! the parenting books said. *Not everyone bonds right away.*

And then she arrived. Checked in at 9½ pounds, 21 inches. *Big baby! Picture of health! Now there's a pair of lungs!*

When the delivery room nurse placed the wailing bundle into my arms, I looked down into her face and said her name. She stopped crying and went very still, as if she were listening.

"She knows who you are," said the nurse.

I felt rapture, then. And deep, deep love. It was immediate and it was forever.

I breastfed for a year, and when I stopped, it was gradual, what happened to Caitlin: digestive problems, weight loss, pale, salty skin, cold after cold. But what did I know? Humans sweat salt. Babies caught colds. I didn't know how unusual it was to have a never-ending course of them, nor how abnormal was skin so salty it could fade clothing and bedding.

Then the first pneumonia, and *Ow, ow, ow, the way they have to strap her arms up over her head in the wheeled contraption that otherwise looks like a baby walker, her eyes terrified and begging as we leave her alone to be X-rayed.*

That X-ray seemed like the worst thing that could ever happen.

After one hospitalization, there was another, a hospital crib-tent filled with airway-opening mist. Then a trip to Boston Children's Hospital to "rule out cystic fibrosis." I had heard of cystic fibrosis at a college fundraiser and all I remembered about it was the weird, ugly name.

She was diagnosed with the genetic lung disease on her second birthday. CF is caused by a malfunctioning gene, but in 1985, that gene had not yet been identified. All of our questions were answered with some version of "We don't really know."

What was known: CF causes a salt imbalance in the body, which mainly affects mucus-producing organs such as lungs and the pancreas. Healthy lungs are slippery, sterile. CF lungs are sticky and harbor bacteria, which cause infections, which slowly render lung tissue nonfunctioning.

She could live a long life or she could die by Christmas, said the CF fellow who was assigned to talk to Nick and me after the diagnosis. "We don't really know."

He was young and brand new at this, and so nervous that he tittered when he spoke.

That night, Nick went back to his office after the dinner we could not eat. I didn't yet know it but his life purpose, that day, had narrowed, become singular: to make sure his daughter would never have to worry about health care, medical bills, nourishment, comforts.

I read her to sleep, our usual ritual. She was wearing soft, pale-green pajamas, and I tried to speak in my normal bedtime voice but it kept cracking. She had never seen me like this and her smile grew nervous, like the doctor's. She tried to fix the situation. She was still in a crib and stood up to reach my cheek, to pat it and tell me, "It's okay."

❧

I have always kept detailed journals so it is easy, now, so many years later, to sit on the floor of my office and page through those early days. To read about the grief so heavy it hurt to breathe. The inability to speak. To remember that I truly believed we could not possibly ever be happy again.

Now I look to find the mistakes we might have made, innocent mistakes made at the very beginning, those first two years when those baby lungs were still healthy and pink and so vulnerable, small as tiny Seckel pears.

The nursery vaporizer I used, only because my mother had always used one. Needlessly promoting bacterial growth.

Baby powder, the particles that must have made their way into her lungs.

Visiting relatives and friends who smoked. Smoking restaurants, taxis, nonsmoking sections on airplanes just seats away from rows of people puffing away. The smoke so thick and stinging, one time, that I had to ask the flight attendant for a cup of ice and hold it to our eyes.

❦

From childhood I have been obsessed with the mystery of our existence within time.

Now my obsession intensifies. I keep thinking that time will go backward, or forward in a different way, that I *will* see her again. She's mine, she's familiar, I know every inch of that face, that face exists, it *must*. How can it not?

Life has become excruciating and heightened and there has been great confusion but also great clarity. When you lose what's most important to you, pretty much everything else falls away and you're left with the fact of yourself, still existing in a world that must make sense if you're to continue living in it.

In a kitchen cabinet, taped to the inside doors, are recipes, poems, cholesterol counts, phone numbers of relatives in Ireland, a Carol Shields quote.

There is a small calendar there, too, that I taped up in early 2014.

I had looked at all the days still to come and wondered what they would bring. Along the bottom I had scribbled, *What will happen???* Knowing there would be an answer, impatient for it.

Now I am impatient for another answer, for the most important answer—what's it all for, what happens when we die, where is she? *Is* she?

Soon after the CF diagnosis, I'd had to travel way out to the Catskills for an overnight business meeting. It was held at one of those sprawling old resort hotels like the one portrayed in *Dirty Dancing*.

That night, in my room at the Mohonk Mountain House, I turned off the bedside lamp and tumbled into a blackness so thick not a single photon of light reached my eyes, no matter how wide I tried to open them. All of the separate worries and fears that routinely flickered through my consciousness became singular, chest-crushing. My life had gone terribly off-path. I had planned to write fiction that readers would find meaningful and I was writing technical manuals instead. I had not planned on children and now I was mother to a child doctors said could worsen and die at any time.

Life had never been so uncertain nor so precious.

That night, the recognition that we all would certainly cease to exist, a reality that I had always accepted with a certain agnostic's resignation, terrified me.

She could not cease to exist.

Not then. Not till later, as we all would, someday so far off in the distant future that it would never really arrive, or when it did, we would already be so old we would be ready.

A sense of resolve filled my life. CF kids were advised to do chest physical therapy every day. To loosen the mucus in the lungs, to encourage coughing, to try to keep bacteria from colonizing in the airways. I vowed to never miss a day, and never did.

Nutrition awareness wasn't yet in the forefront of our culture, but we had Bread & Circus, a local organic grocery store chain that Whole Foods would one day gobble up. It only made sense that a nourished body must fare better. I fed that two-year-old so well that she became a four-year-old who one day astonished a fellow shopper by jumping up and down in the produce aisle, begging for *broccoli! broccoli!*

She knew she had CF like she knew she had teeth in her mouth. She brushed her teeth. She took her meds; put up with the daily, half-hour-long treatments of chest PT, which we attempted to turn into fun by calling them "tap tap"; went into the hospital for two-week courses of intravenous antibiotic therapy—called "cleanouts"—when necessary.

She's so stoic, people said.

She was. I watched her in tense situations—blood draws, blood gas tests, IV-line insertions—the way she focused inwardly and became calm. She expressed her fears in private ways.

One night, I heard her in her bed, talking to herself. "Always have to cough, don't know why."

I found little drawings.

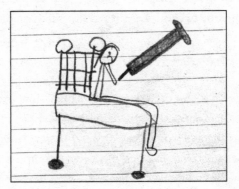

And I lived in the moment.

I lived in the moment.

I put CF in a box.

And lived in the moment.

Eased now, by the balm of passed time, is the pain of moments lived inside that box. The fear when a crisis reared and we had to cancel everything and pack our bags for two weeks in the hospital. Watching heavy-duty meds infuse into baby veins. Three-times-a-day chest PT pounding. It didn't seem possible that a body could withstand all that. And always, the suppressed panic, the waiting for results, praying she would get back to her baseline.

She always did get better. And discoveries felt rapid, those early years. Within months of her diagnosis, a DNA marker linked to CF was reported to be on chromosome 7. And when she was six, scientists finally discovered the "CF gene"—a gene responsible for chloride-transport function. Mutations of that gene caused the disease known as CF. Now gene therapy was not only possible, but also likely.

I knew we couldn't sit around and wait—or worse, *trust* that it would happen, but gene therapy was part of that big shining orb of hope for the future, and we had a job to do: keep her well so that when gene therapy became a reality, she would benefit.

Tap tap tap tap tap, tap tap tap tap tap. Long, slow exhale, to clear the airways. *Tap tap tap tap tap, tap tap tap tap tap.*

Each morning at six o'clock, Caitlin's physical therapist lets herself in, tiptoes upstairs, and begins doing tap tap on a half-asleep Caitlin.

On this particular morning, the one I am reliving through an old, detailed diary entry, I will be driving Caitlin to a new school. Once we realized that she and another girl in her third-grade class were being given busywork—stapling worksheet packets while the teacher worked with children who needed help—we applied to a local private school known for its small classes, supportive family atmosphere, and overall excellence in academics, art, and sports.

During the interviews, we downplayed her cystic fibrosis. The school was upfront about not being equipped for children who had special needs. And Caitlin didn't—generally. Cleanouts were once or twice a year and we had learned that we could, once she had an IV line placed, infuse the meds at home with an on-call nurse on board to change dressings and draw blood labs.

This September morning, she eats her breakfast, takes her digestive enzymes and her daily assortment of antibiotics, her inhaler and nasal steroid spray. Then I drive her the twelve minutes to the school. She is confident and expectant, wondering aloud what the first day will be like, and I am thankful for her natural social poise, which always makes life easier.

I am a new student, too. After my night in the Mohonk Mountain House, I declared myself to be in early midlife crisis and enrolled in a graduate writing program in Boston. Twice a week I immerse myself, finally, in the world of letters I've longed for.

Late that afternoon, I pick her up. We have the first version of the conversation we will have for the next ten years.

"How was your day?"

"Great."

"Tell me about it."

"I liked my teachers. The history teacher, especially. And I really like this girl Kenley. She invited me to her house on Saturday."

Kenley would become, like many in that school, the closest kind of lifelong friend.

And I would write, in these pages I now clutch to my chest: *Normal life is happening. We have some control over this.*

❦

Fay School was in Southborough, a town adjacent to ours, and over the years I usually took one of two routes to drive there. At a certain point along Route 85, we encountered a fork. I could choose to go right, up and down over a long hilly road, or left, which wound around the flat of the hill. Both roads took the same amount of time. I never decided until I reached the fork.

One morning, a car sat within the fork, at the stop sign. I clearly had the right of way, no matter which way I decided to go, but I had decided to go left. I did not need an indicator because left was technically straight.

As we were almost upon the car, right in the crosshairs of the intersection, the driver pulled out. I braked so hard that I rose out of my seat.

We were rattled but unharmed. Close calls like this happened every once in a while, to everyone. But as I continued the drive to school, I thought of the what-ifs and I looked over at Caitlin, who was in fourth grade by then. I was thirty-four. We were so close. She called us "mostly companions" and I reveled in her existence. Our present seemed like it must last forever. But I thought about how even if we lived long lives, "long lives" only meant another forty or so years together. This was not forever.

❦

Keeping CF lungs undamaged was a hard battle. CF is a progressive disease, and cruel in its invisibility. CF people look so normal, and deterioration can be so gradual, that bad news can come at you overnight. Like the need for the lobectomy when she was eleven.

During a "normal" pulmonary exacerbation, her cystic fibrosis team discovered that a slow-growing, stealthy mycobacterium (MAI) had destroyed the lower lobe of her left lung. Left unchecked, the MAI would spread to the other two left lobes, and then into her right lung.

The only way to save her was with major thoracic surgery that would cut away the ruined lobe and hopefully stop the spread.

Lobectomy. Frankenstein language.

Just a week before this news, the three of us had easily climbed a small mountain in New Hampshire, Caitlin as able as any other kid on the trail. I was finishing my last year of my writing program and it had gone so well. I'd met people I knew would be life friends. An editor at *The New Yorker* was actively encouraging my submissions. That night in our rental cabin, I had let myself hope: *Maybe we will be able to live normally! Maybe Caitlin will be one of those mostly unaffected CF people who grow old uneventfully!* We knew some of them. A man who was almost sixty. A runner who was in her thirties—both of them diagnosed at a time when CF life expectancy was in the single digits.

And now the Fates had punished me for my attempt at denial. For trying to escape my path and will an easier one into being.

During those days leading up to the March surgical date, I tried to focus on my thesis—a story collection—due, also, in March, but I was terrified for all the reasons a parent is terrified when a child needs surgery. Compounding the fear was that the outcome was not certain. The thoracic team wouldn't know until they got inside and actually saw her lungs whether the mycobacteria's spread could indeed be stopped.

When she was at school and Nick was at his office and I was

alone in the house, I did things like cling to doorjambs and scream. I lay on my living room sofa and sobbed.

I was on that sofa one bright winter morning when I heard a voice. Strong and quite clear, a low female voice. It said, *Have faith*.

I sat up. I blinked and looked around at the furniture, the bookshelves, the windows and doors.

I thought about how easy it would be to doubt what I had heard.

⁂

Much of her memory of that time would be clouded by painkillers, but Caitlin remembered waking in the dimly lit ICU and hearing that the damaged lobe was gone, that the rest of her lungs looked clear and healthy. She remembered the pinches of multiple IV lines in her arms and legs, the chest tubes sutured into her torso. The tubes drained leaking fluids into plastic receptacles. They would remain in place for a week or two until the lung repaired itself.

Except . . . the lung did not repair itself. Oh, the tubes were removed and we were discharged home, expectations being that she would soon be her normal self.

But recovery didn't progress as predicted. One day, I looked out an upstairs window and saw her in the yard, clenching her fists and running back and forth as fast she could, trying to improve her lung function.

In May, I graduated from my MFA program. She was in the audience with Nick, her face so gaunt and skeletal but beaming when I received the Graduate Dean's Award, which pleased me primarily because it felt so important to be an inspiration to her, my girl child.

That night, we stayed in a Boston hotel to celebrate, and the generous hotel upgraded us to a suite. At 3:00 a.m., Nick and I woke to strange, periodic huffing sounds coming from beyond the bedroom wall. They were coming from her.

Back in the hospital at first light, we waited for the X-ray results. The three of us, tight within our bodies, braced ourselves for the news we knew had to be bad. And it was. Air leaking from her lung had created a pneumothorax—air in the chest—so large it had pushed aside her heart.

Her surgical team reinserted the chest tubes, this time attaching them to a suctioning device behind her hospital bed, to keep a steady vacuum pressure on the lung to keep it inflated and help it drain.

But the lung did not heal. Her surgeon speculated that perhaps they had not completely removed all the damaged tissue. After a week, she underwent the thoracic surgery a second time. But once inside, everything looked clear.

Weeks passed as she lay trapped in that bed, attached to the vacuum. We canceled the summer adventure in Paris that was to have been the lobectomy's reward. From her ninth-floor room, we could see ball games at Fenway Park, and one night, Fourth of July fireworks. We began to know nurses by their knock. Junk mail from takeout food companies would be delivered to us in the regular mail. Nick popped in when he could but spent most of his time growing his company, taking on ever bigger jobs, building a reputation for integrity and workmanship, always conscious of the door-knocking wolf that was the expensive health care Caitlin would forever need.

A team of infectious disease specialists from Boston Children's and Brigham and Women's hospitals tried to figure out why she was not healing. No one could come up with anything more than a speculative theory. Every few days, the team would check, via X-ray, whether the air was still leaking. It always was, and her eyes began to lose their light. Years later she would write about that time:

> *When I was 11, I was very sick for a long time, and I had a hospital physical therapist who would come in and do chest PT. She would talk about God and Jesus, almost in an awkwardly preachy way . . . she was Southern. But I was so sick and so detached from anything normal that an 11-year-old kid thinks about, that I just fell into it. And she encouraged me to pray and so I did, and I prayed a lot all through my teenage years. And I can still remember her talking to me as I stared out the window and I can't believe that was an 11-year-old kid. It was like I stopped being a kid that year.*

Boston Children's Hospital offered the staff of brilliant nurses, doctors, and various therapists one expects. It also offered something rare: a spacious and magical healing garden—a private park, really, with a broad lawn and meandering paths—tucked deep inside the center of the hospital's sundry, cobbled-together-over-time buildings.

Olive Higgins Prouty, a Boston author and philanthropist, had lost two young daughters to illness and, in the 1950s, endowed, in perpetuity, a garden for children. She hired the famous Olmsted Brothers to design the space, but requested that it appear natural, so that sick children could truly experience nature.

Green grass. Hide-and-seek bushes. Bunnies. Dirt and bright flowers and a shallow pool that welcomed ducks. A rare dawn redwood tree, sixty-five feet tall, with a thick red trunk, sheltering limbs, and deep roots.

To give Caitlin a break, her team began to temporarily remove her from the wall suction and attach the chest tubes to receptacles that a nurse and I could carry so she could walk, or travel in a wheelchair, to this one place of light and grace that she was able to experience during those months we waited for that lung to heal.

We picnicked there, and some days Nick brought in lacrosse sticks and the two of them tossed the ball back and forth. I have many garden memories, but the image that is foremost is of Caitlin's small self, standing with her head tilted back, long rubber tubing connecting her chest to drain boxes that sit on the ground by her feet. Her gaze is skyward, she is happy, taking in the vast height, the presence of that majestic dawn redwood.

That tree was always her favorite part of the Prouty Garden.

For this mother, the most comforting thing was the plaque at its entrance: *The garden will continue to exist at Children's Hospital as long as there are patients, families, and staff to enjoy it.*

❦

My stack of journals is full of the details that sum up those years after the surgery and all its complications. The *will-the-MAI-come-back?* anxiety. CT scans replacing routine lung X-rays. The hospital's world-renowned chief pulmonologist, the brilliant Mary Ellen Wohl, saying she would take over as Caitlin's personal doctor because "Caitlin can't have a doctor who thinks within the rules."

> **May 6, 1999** *CT scan. 1% area of granular nodules, spot on left and spot on right.*
>
> *Starting another 6 weeks of IV clarithromycin, ethambutol, and cipro.*
>
> *Please please please let this work to keep her lungs clear.*

Six weeks on IVs were tough but they were six-week courses we could do mainly at home: get the IV line in at the hospital, sign for the cartons of meds and syringes and saline and heparin the home care company delivered to the house. A nurse once a week to draw labs and change the dressing that hid under a normal sleeve of clothing. Round-the-clock, two-hour infusions, the worst at 1:00 a.m. because Caitlin didn't trust anyone to administer her meds and sat up to ensure no mistakes. Because mistakes happened all the time, even in places like Boston Children's Hospital, and she learned that lesson early and well.

The medications were strong. They filled her with nausea and drained her energy reserves, but home cleanouts let her go to school and live somewhat normally when she would otherwise have had to be hospitalized.

All those crises. So much underlying worry. *What if she doesn't bounce back? What if she gets so sick we have to go back into the hospital only this time we never get out and what if what if what if?*

But there was determination, too. I vowed to do everything I could to control her health and keep her well, and all our efforts seemed to work. A couple of years passed. CF slowly went back into its box.

High school: her wilder, rebellious side gleefully flouted the sillier rules at her traditional New England prep school. She met Jess and others who became lifelong friends, and found her passion in the writings of Virginia Woolf and in AP art history classes. "I'm so lucky to have found out what I love, so early," she told me.

March 15, 2000 *Caitlin was accepted at GW, and was offered their art history merit scholarship, worth 50 percent of tuition. Amazing and totally unexpected! She really wants to go there. Wants urban.*

We dropped her off at college. Her dorm was two blocks from the White House, as urban as she had wanted. She had chosen a six-person unit so she could see what it was like, as an only child, to live with others.

Wow. It's really happening. She's living normally. We were choked up leaving DC, but by the time we crossed the George Washington Bridge, Nick and I were realizing we finally had the together time we never got to experience as expectant newlyweds. We discovered a fun little Mexican cantina on the Connecticut border where we ordered taquitos and raised our margaritas and let ourselves believe that everything might very well be okay.

September 11, 2001 *Finally got hold of Caitlin at 11:30. She said it's chaos there, no one knows what's going on. She can see the Pentagon burning from her window.*

Weeks later came the first of the 2001 anthrax attacks. And then we were into sophomore year and the DC area began to experience three weeks of terror from a random sniper. On Parents' Weekend, we arrived on a Thursday evening to deserted streets. In the lobby on Friday morning, the hotel's televisions broadcast news of the latest killing, of a man pumping gas on a highway in Virginia.

And then she got sick. Older parents had warned us that college could be a dangerous time, when CF kids often lived in denial of their fragile health, and Caitlin was no different. At midterm she got so sick that we saw that the CF support system I had set up in DC was as flimsy as I had prayed it would not be. She flew home after exams and checked in to Children's for a cleanout. The staff immediately put her on hospital precautions, everyone entering her room required to wear gowns, gloves, masks. But why? A nurse casually informed us that her lungs were culturing that organism that only 3 percent of CF patients ever culture but that everyone dreads and is sometimes associated with rapid decline and death and that is always associated with increased decline: *Burkholderia cepacia* had been colonizing in her lungs for two years, there had been some kind of breakdown in communication with new hospital record-keeping software combined with Caitlin's out-of-town status and Dr. Wohl's retirement, and *what the hell was happening?*

I tried to hide my terror. This was like everything else, I said aloud to her. Cepacia affected everyone differently. We would do everything we could to fight it.

But *cepacia*.

She flew back to DC to take her finals. And began to arrange a transfer to a Boston school.

3

THE BOX

One day I arrived for an appointment of my own. The receptionist put away her book, but I asked what she was reading. I'm always curious.

"A book about past lives." She noted my skepticism and clarified: *This* particular author had real-world credentials. He was a psychiatrist named Brian Weiss, an MD and PhD with degrees from Columbia and Yale. Former head of psychiatry at Miami's Mount Sinai. He had come very reluctantly and unexpectedly to the practice of past life regression.

Those facts intrigued me, and later I would wonder if I had been led to that book—for comfort, at the very least. I read Dr. Weiss's book and found his story compelling. If you believed this man—and that was key, of course, but he came across as genuine—then his message was kind of irrefutable: that we are essentially souls who lead many lives.

I did a little more reading—about Dr. Ian Stevenson, another psychiatrist who had been conducting methodical reincarnation research, for decades, at the University of Virginia School of

Medicine. I was intrigued by these dry, meticulous case studies of researchers attempting, often unsuccessfully, to disconfirm paranormal explanations for children's past-life stories. I remembered, too, the odd things kids sometimes said, like the time my friend's three-year-old casually said to my friend, "Remember when I was your mother?"

I was drawn to the idea of the evolution and growth of the soul. It seemed to me to be the only thing that made sense of human suffering. It also supported the argument that humanity is essentially good.

I gifted the Weiss book to Caitlin. She had had a fairly stable couple of years, living on her own, interning at the Isabella Stewart Gardner Museum, attending Boston College. She and I had even managed a couple of trips that we miraculously did not have to cancel—Italy one summer, an apartment in Paris the next spring, but infections were becoming more frequent. She didn't bounce back to baseline after cleanouts. Instead her pulmonary function test numbers mostly and slowly declined.

I hoped the book would help to allay the fear that was surely inside her.

❦

She was home for the night, in her childhood bedroom, not sick enough for IV meds but not feeling well, either. I was awake in the night, sitting up in the dark, going over my concerns in my head.

When you're desperate, you will try anything.

I thought of the occasional times she and I had experienced powerful energy exchanges—volt-like, palpable currents we could actually feel and sometimes hear.

I slipped out of bed to position my body to face the direction of her room and, by force of will, imagined cleansing energy pass through her, head to toe.

Then I went back to bed and forgot about it.

In the morning, she slept very late. When she came downstairs, she looked at me strangely. "Did you do something last night?"

"Why?"

"I woke up and there was all this white at the foot of my bed. I coughed and coughed and cleared so much that I slept all the way till now."

Of course there were plenty of times I tried such things and nothing happened. The difference was that the successful times would be accompanied by a strong sense of connecting and of *knowing* that I was connecting. A kind of certainty.

※

For years, Caitlin had longed for a little dog and tried to pester me into getting one. "What's wrong with you?" she would say, utterly exasperated with me. "You could have any little pup you want!"

I didn't want to be tied down any more than I already was.

But in Ireland, where Nick grew up and where his whole family lived, turning twenty-one was a big deal. Celebrations were similar to bat mitzvahs and *quinceañeras*. Caitlin knew she could ask for pretty much anything the year she turned twenty-one.

She was in the middle of a home cleanout, IV line and bandage concealed beneath her sweatshirt when we visited the breeder and she chose a quiet little Yorkshire terrier male. She had decided she would call him Henry, although when she discovered he was born on February 2, Groundhog Day, she half considered Phil.

Groundhog Day was a favorite family movie, always good for jokes and laughs. The delightful fact of his birthday "sealed the deal," she said.

Nick hadn't been keen on paying money for a dog—the very idea, when he was growing up in Ireland, would have been unimaginable—but as we stood in the breeder's kitchen, he softened. He always softens. Who wouldn't? Caitlin's face was so lit with joy, the little pup tucked into the crook of her arm. Henry was painfully adorable: pointy ears and black button eyes, little pink tongue.

I remembered Hobo, my beloved childhood dog. Coming home from first grade to the news that he had been hit by a car. That first bout with unbearable grief. Scrambling to write a little book about him, stapling the pages together, book-making the only thing that made me feel better. The simple declarative sentences. *Hobo, he was a good dog.*

She was already in love. I knew I was going to fall in love, too, even as I tried to protect myself. *That dog has a longer life expectancy than your daughter.*

I hoped I was wrong.

In the summer of 2005, she was admitted to the hospital for the second time that year. The first morning, as always, I cooked her day's meals at home, then headed into Boston.

I knocked on her door and walked in but she wasn't herself. She was sitting up very straight in the bed, edgy, irritable. Finally she admitted what was wrong. "So they want me to go on the transplant list."

I was aware of dividing in two: a sense of myself falling to the ground as I spoke with calm concern. "What did they say?"

"They actually said it last time I was in. But I didn't tell anyone, and now they're talking again."

"You've been holding this in this whole time?" I moved to hug her, but she jerked away.

"Do NOT feel sorry for me. I didn't tell anyone because I want people to want to BE me, not feel sorry for me."

Which made me smile and saved me from losing it. Such a fireball.

I stayed in mother mode and faked strength and confidence, the way we parents do, but I was choking on grief. She was so beautiful and smart and fiery, the invisibility of CF both a gift and a curse. Just that day someone had said, the way people said all the time, *Caitlin looks great!*

She would look great for the rest of her life.

<hr />

On September 1, 2005, I wrote, *A heart-heavy day. Admitted, 3rd time this year, 2nd time in three months. She's sad and scared.*

Transplant evaluation, a lengthy process made up of multiple appointments, was due to start. She had an IV line placed at the hospital, then I moved into her apartment to help her with the meds, the dog, all of it, so she could still go to school.

To minimize walking, I drove her to her classes and picked her up afterward. One day she told me it embarrassed her to take the elevator from the first floor to the second. "I look normal and people get really pissed off, so today when the door opened, I limped off."

We laughed about that. It became one of those family jokes that you shorthand and repeat, the kind of joke that keeps you close and keeps you laughing.

Dumb jokes become hilarious because they're a release valve. Chronic anxiety is part of chronic illness. When you're waiting for results, for improvements, you are forced to wait through time—days, hours, weeks, months. Laughter helps.

At the end of two such weeks, her pulmonary function tests had gone down ten points. A CT scan showed new, small, all-over areas of infection. She was nauseated and weak and coughing up blood. I was terrified. Medicine had never before not helped, and now, with our beloved Dr. Wohl retired, I felt adrift. The new doctor kept stressing that weight gain was critical.

At home I finally said, "Look. This is basic stuff. We can at least get you to gain weight." I calculated how many calories her body, in its constant state of inflammation, likely burned, and developed a plan. A plan to strictly record food intake and to drink thousand-calorie, nourishing shakes twice a day.

***

September 14, 2005 *Weird thing last night. We'd left the TV on by mistake. I got up to get the 1AM meds and a TV station was playing a show about George Washington's church in New York City. I heard Caitlin get up and looked into the living room to see what was happening. She was in the bathroom throwing up, and on the TV, the words to the Hail Mary prayer were starting to scroll. Then a simple, "Trust God."*

Caitlin's always had an affinity for Mary.

We look for signs, don't we? For assurance, for some kind of sense.

***

Like all lives, ours has had its dividing lines, its befores and afters, but one of the toughest was the October day when Caitlin's doctor said she needed to start using supplemental oxygen for sleeping and for flying—those times when everyone's oxygen saturation levels naturally go down, but go down more dramatically, and dangerously, when you have lung disease.

The need for oxygen was a game-changer. The concentrator weighed forty pounds and had to be plugged in. It wasn't something you could bring onto a plane. The other option, portable tanks, were heavy and needed to be frequently refilled.

Traveling, always our salvation and reward, was going to be difficult.

As always, I scrambled for things to be optimistic about. The calorie-counting was going well. The twice-a-day thousand-calorie shakes.

And her doctor was going to try something new, a shot in the dark. Something some cystic fibrosis teams in Denmark were doing with good results. Mixing ceftazidime, which is usually delivered intravenously, and putting it into a nebulizer. Inhaling it for a half hour twice a day.

※

October 22, 2005 *So: Caitlin looks wonderful! I feared I was just being hopeful but everyone can see a difference. She is off the IVs and she weighs 104.5 pounds! Ten pounds in less than four weeks!*

When I picked her up last night, she said that the inhaled ceftaz has "given her a new lease on life." That it no longer takes her all day to clear her lungs and feel well, and that she no longer has to stop and rest on her way to class. The other day she was doing laundry and ran up and down the stairs rather than wait for the elevator.

After just a week on the inhaled ceftaz, Caitlin had felt well enough that I had been able to resume my normal life at home. I even planned a mother/daughter weekend in Vermont with my best friend and her daughter Katie, Caitlin's oldest friend, who had been in England for the past year, studying for a master's degree at Cambridge University.

Katie: Born nine months before Caitlin, she came into my life just as I was grappling with the reality of my unplanned pregnancy. Falling in love with her calmed some of my maternal fears, and from the beginning, she and Caitlin grew up, essentially, as sisters.

There exists an old snapshot of first-grade Katie, getting off the school bus, that is like a blueprint for how she's lived her life. The camera's caught her in midair, flying off the bus steps, arms spread wide, full of excitement and anxious to share every detail of her day. Caitlin had missed Katie terribly, and it felt important to be able to do a fun, normal trip like this. I strapped the forty-pound concentrator into the back seat of our car like a passenger. Then I hauled that passenger into the inn, pretending to myself that travel was still completely doable. And it was, sort of.

But the next morning in Vermont, I woke up early. She looked so young and small, asleep, the plastic cannula on her face.

I watched her and wrote, *I don't know what to pray for anymore.* She obviously had worsening lung damage, needed oxygen, and was going to need a transplant at some point. But now, miraculously, transplant could be put off, and hopefully for a long, long time. *I hope she will find her purpose*, I wrote.

A couple of years after I discovered the Brian Weiss book, I saw that he was going to be doing an event in Massachusetts.

I wanted to see him in person, and wanted to take Caitlin. But it was a gamble. If he wasn't for real, I would just *know*. And so would she.

We were both wary but open. The more serious UVA-type reincarnation research impressed Caitlin, and with a bit of be-mused distance—it was all still speculative then, nothing was yet at stake—we had begun to explore more of this metaphysical stuff. She stumbled into an experience with a self-described soul reader, who gave her such an uncanny reading, anonymously, and from afar, that I broke into goose bumps and cried listening to her recount it.

We also became interested in astrology, not the sun sign horo-scope in a newspaper type of astrology but the complicated chart of energy configurations of planets and star positions that suppos-edly influences you like a thumbprint when you are born. There are plenty of naysayers who make good points, and I don't know of anyone who can explain why there really seems to be something to it. But there just is. Even when the broadest of brushstrokes are painted, there is *no* mistaking an Aries male for a Libran. Caitlin and I even got to the point where we could be watching *60 Minutes*, see a guy interviewed, and say, O my God, he's such a Cancer. And we'd Google and be right.

The Weiss event was held at a hotel where the doctor spoke to a room of about two hundred of us. He was as I had imagined him to be: a gentle man with a kind, soft-spoken manner. Honestly, he was a tiny bit boring. But I welcomed that. He was no showman with tricks. I was relieved.

After his talk, he told us that he was going to do a couple of group regressions—hypnosis to help the mind work backward. He explained how he would conduct them; then the room went dim and quiet. He led us all into a light hypnotic trance state. I was interrupted by an itch and lost my focus, but Caitlin easily reached a thetaish state and over lunch reported three vivid experiences to me, the details of which I scribbled down so we wouldn't forget.

When she looked over the notes, she said it was wild how much they resonated with feelings she'd always had inside. Still, "It doesn't prove anything," she said. "I could have invented it all."

But Weiss also led another group exercise. He first explained that most people possess unrecognized, untapped intuitive abilities. Then he had us exchange personal items with a stranger, hold them and reflect on them, then write down whatever came to mind, with no hesitation or censoring. I had an accurate exchange with my stranger, as did Caitlin, and as she said herself, "I couldn't have invented any of that."

Caitlin had held her stranger's wedding and engagement rings. She recounted:

> First I saw a ferry, an ocean. Then a sailboat. The ocean was New England or mid-Atlantic. My first thought was "Maine," then "No, maybe Rhode Island. Lower than Massachusetts. Rhode Island seems right."
>
> My next thought was "Franklin," then I focused on the "N." And that the rings seemed associated with a lengthy period of time. I thought: "It took a long time to get these rings."

The stranger was a woman married to a sailor who wore his uniform at their wedding in the shore town of Narragansett, Rhode Island, after a very long engagement.

The second half of the Brian Weiss day was another group event, led by a medium named John Holland. We didn't plan to stay—we didn't trust that what we might see would be anything but cold reading—but in the end decided to stick around and observe for the heck of it.

John Holland's performance was impressive, but . . . I'd once had a professional Las Vegas magician do incredible card tricks right in front of my eyes.

Then, about an hour into the event, he looked over toward the general area where Caitlin and I were sitting and said he had a message for "Mo, Maureen, name like that" from an older man, father figure, but someone who'd passed fairly young.

I froze. John's voice and manner changed as he went on, "Haha, this guy's a real guinea." "A real guinea" was something my Italian father, Vito, always called himself. Then John did a fist-pump, boxing kind of move that was also a ringer for something my father used to do.

Caitlin dug her nails into my hand. We looked at each other. It was like Vito had taken over John's body in that brief instant. *Raise your hand*, I thought, *this is for you*. But I was still frozen, and during my hesitation a man I had earlier overheard say he was really hoping for a reading "claimed" the spirit and was trying to make everything John said fit. The details did not fit the man, and eventually John moved on, but everything John had said *did* fit me. The one thing I wasn't sure of was that the father wanted to let the audience member's sister know that everything was going to be okay.

The next day I called my sister. She is a registered nurse and quite practical and I thought she would likely scoff at my story, but she surprised me by breaking into tears. "That was for me," she said. "I have no doubt."

She had been having serious problems with her middle daughter and had been in her rocking chair holding our father's watch just days before, asking him to look out for them.

⬧

As with the soul books, I study these old journals of mine, eager to discover assurances that *Yes, the unexplained really did happen. Consciousness might possibly exist apart from the physical.* But I read with an eye that is colder, more suspicious than the bemused, entertained me who originally wrote the records.

In 2006, Caitlin's doctor wanted her to do a cleanout but my instinct told me she just needed the seacoast this time—she needed lots of sleep and some nourishing food and to breathe in some briny ocean air.

And I needed to write. During the past few years I had done so much research for a novel that I hadn't done much writing of it, and that made me anxious.

We stayed in a little hotel in Gloucester, in a room that overlooked a rocky stretch of navy blue Atlantic.

It was one of those weeks that would be remembered as an idyll—mainly because the plan worked. She improved without needing antibiotics.

She rested so deeply on that shore that the first of many occurrences of an occasional odd event happened on the third night there. A strange noise woke me. She was sound asleep but her oxygen tubing was rat-tat-tatting against the end table, rhythmically and fast. The machine hummed as usual. It was not vibrating. But the vibrating tubing noise went on for a while. Then it stopped.

In the morning, she said, "Something really weird happened last night. It sounds crazy but it was like an out-of-body experience."

She said that her body had begun to vibrate and that as she began to move out of it, her first thought was, *Oh, it's just that thing.*

As in, *Don't worry. This is something familiar that you've experienced before.*

Then her more conscious self thought, *Wait! What thing? This is nothing I've experienced before.* And she startled herself out of the state, whatever it was.

She read up on sleep paralysis and learned about vivid hallucinations, called *hypnagogic*, which can appear during the transition from sleep to wakefulness and which the mind perceives as reality, but she was never entirely sure what was really happening when "that thing" happened, as it did many times over the years to come. She never really got over being slightly afraid of it.

⁕

Oh, that sad cartoon image from my own childhood: the frog in the slowly boiling water, adapting, adapting—*It's not that bad . . . No, I'm okay . . . Well, I guess it IS getting a little hot in here . . .*

Her twenties. Declining lung function. Supplemental oxygen. On the surface, still living a normal life, but adapting, adapting. Working in an art gallery on Charles Street, parties, boyfriends, nights at the Sail Loft with her friends, travel. Well enough to forgo the oxygen on nights when it wasn't convenient. Over the years, we had canceled so many vacations that we always held our breath until the plane touched down, and probably canceled one of every four trips we ever planned. But she got in plenty during her twenties: family trips to St. John, to Europe. Spring break trips with her friends. Mother-daughter adventures. A father-daughter trip to the West of Ireland.

The third-floor walkup with parking a quarter mile down the street becomes impossible, so you move to a building with an elevator. Problem solved, until the twenty-seven steps from the street parking—if you find a spot—to the lobby, to the elevator, become the next impossible. So you move to a building with an elevator, no stairs, indoor parking.

You adapt. That's what we humans do. We're coded to adapt.

Still, all the while, as the mother, you see that this age really is, as they warned you, the most painful time to watch your child live with a disease.

Caitlin's friends—they were all living with the same physical freedom I took for granted when I lived in Ireland and dated Nick. Kenley at Buzzfeed in New York, Katie getting that first master's at Cambridge, then another in Madrid, Jess discovering an enduring passion for Kenya, Alyssa buying for Bergdorf's in New York, Mieke in London and Paris, and *O my God, Mum, Mieke has the coolest life.*

Adapting continued. As much as she wanted to pursue a graduate degree in philosophy, she realized she needed a career that would let her work at her own pace. She completed a graphic design course, then became the in-house designer for a digital imaging arts school affiliated with Boston University.

One winter, Nick and I had a long-anticipated, three-week trip to the Caribbean planned. A St. John villa, some sailing, then ending on St. Kitts with friends. The night before we were set to leave, she called, apologizing. Her fever was 101 and rising.

A virus that a healthy human can endure can be lethal for a compromised person. That morning, we were in the ER with her, canceling flights and hotels. A more brutal than normal cleanout began.

As her lung function declined, her CF team once again encouraged her to get going on the extensive series of lung transplant evaluation appointments at Brigham and Women's Hospital. To be on the safe side. To be evaluated and accepted, not necessarily actively listed.

That way, if your health suddenly went south, you would be all set.

As one transplant coordinator once told Caitlin, *Oh, honey, hang on to your native lungs for as long as you can.*

A transplant can be confusing for people who are healthy and have the true luxury of taking good health for granted. On the surface, a transplant can seem like an easy fix, but replacing a major organ in one's body is as serious as it gets. There are risks throughout the entire process—the surgery, the recovery, the aftermath.

Here's an exercise:

Put a straw into your mouth and seal your lips around it, tightly. Plug up your nostrils with some duct tape. Now, breathing only through that straw, climb a nearby hill. Then go to the grocery store, or go to work. Take a shower. Go out to dinner. Keep getting all your air from that straw.

Okay, now imagine that your once-pink lungs are so black and charred and crusty and useless that there is no way you can continue to live with them and that feeble little straw in your mouth.

Your only hope is to be the recipient of someone else's worst misfortune.

Because both lungs are diseased by the time you need a transplant, both must be removed and replaced with two healthy lungs. Two are necessary because leaving an empty space inside the chest would leave you at risk for infection.

It's the most major kind of surgery, with a recovery involving the most intense kind of pain.

Okay, you say. You can live through that. Because the end result is worth it, which it is.

But now your body, posttransplant, says, *I don't recognize these foreign objects, even though they are keeping me alive. I will reject them.*

So your immune system needs to be repressed.

No one needs to be told about how hard it is to live with no immune system. Forever after, you will have to live with a level of care and caution that you never before had to give a thought to.

So. You don't want a transplant until your quality of life is poor. Still, you must be healthy enough to survive the major surgery.

Transplant timing is one of those "fine lines."

Caitlin began to schedule the evaluation appointments. There were many. Ventilation perfusion scans, CT scans, pulmonary function tests, tissue typing, EKGs, blood tests, mental health workups, emotional support determinations.

But her experience with the transplant team was chaotic from the start. Their evaluation procedure was unstructured, done piecemeal. She showed up for more than one appointment that she had scheduled but no one had recorded, and was sent home.

Months into this erratic process, a shock. As Caitlin would write in a letter to Vertex Pharmaceuticals in 2011, in a plea for compassionate use of their new gene-modifying drug Kalydeco, in its final trials:

> *Last fall, I underwent transplant evaluation at University of Pittsburgh Medical Center, and was accepted into the program, where I will become listed when the time comes to do so. I felt incredibly positive about my experience at UPMC, and I know I am in a great place. It is not easy though, imagining and then*

undergoing a procedure like a lung transplant outside of one's own home city. UPMC remains my only option for lung transplant at this time, because I am excluded from all other programs due to my having b. Cepacia (cenocepacia). I actually underwent the evaluation process at the Brigham and Women's a few years ago, but after completing two-thirds of it, the committee at BWH decided (like most other clinics during this time) to suspend transplantation of cenocepacia patients. I contracted cepacia while in the hospital when I was 17 years old, so it should come as no surprise that this has been a conflicted and difficult process, mentally as well as physically.

A calm summary that in no way reflected the panic and anguish this brutal decision would eventually cause. But at first, she was mainly perplexed and left me a voice message: "Some random person from the transplant department called and said they're not going to transplant me. Because of my cepacia. And I said, no no. I was so confused. I said you do transplant cepacia. But some study came out and all the hospitals are saying no to cepacia."

We investigated what happened, and yes, it was all because of one old and limited study. The decision was unfair, but all the hospitals were falling in line with it.

Except for Pittsburgh. But what if Pittsburgh decided to stop transplanting cepacia patients, too? My mind began desperate what-if options. Europe? Asia?

Pittsburgh hung over our heads until finally, in 2009, Caitlin made her decision. She would go to Pittsburgh and do the weeklong evaluation in 2010.

From: Caitlin O'Hara
To: Mom
Date: February 9, 2009, 5:02p.m.
Subject: "25 random things about me"

This thing is going around Facebook. I did one but I'm not going to post it.

1.   Sometimes to help me fall asleep I take one sock off with the opposite foot's toe, and then take the other sock off with the other toe, but only halfway and leave my toe in the sock.

2.   I like to eat bread-and-butter chip pickles with pad thai when it's really really hot out and I can't wait to do that this summer.

3.   I would actually like to eat those bugs they fry up that you see on TV in Asia.

4.   I have the tendency to re-read books, listen to songs over and over, and re-watch movies to the point of ridiculousness.

5.   I remember movie lines verbatim, even the pitch of the character's voice.

6.   I think these things are stupid.

7.   One time an escargot slipped out of its pincers up, up into the air, down my shirt, and into my bag in a cafe in Paris while I screamed ahhhh!

8.   I like to take showers in the dark at night before I go out, and in the summertime I will bring a beer in there.

9.   I can't stand the feel of the water that collects in dishes in the dishwasher when it is clean. When that water touches me, I get the shivers.

10. I am not scared of spiders, mice, or snakes. But I am REPULSED by eyes that grow out of potatoes. One time red ones grew out of a sweet potato I had and it sent me into dry heaves.

11. I like to tell jokes in hospitals.

12. I have parking karma. I hope I don't ruin it by stating that.

13. My left breast is bigger than my right. My left is my favorite.

14. I can cross my eyes all different directions but this seems to really disturb some people. I must look really scary when I do it, but I can't see this because my eyes are crossed.

15. I love Cherry Garcia ice cream so much that I had to start buying the frozen yogurt, not because I am afraid of getting fat but because I don't think it is good for one person to consume so many grams of fat and dairy like that.

16. I love looking at myself in the mirror when my hair is in hot rollers.

17. I love looking at myself in the mirror.

18. One of my absolute favorite things to do is just drive around by myself and listen to music. When I go on vacation and don't drive, or am not alone, I feel a real withdrawal from this. I like to cry too when I do this.

19. I love birds, all kinds of birds. I wish it wasn't creepy to own them.

20. I love graveyards and cemeteries, and all my friends who live in them.

21. I love the look of my own handwriting, which I cultivated and intentionally developed in the sixth grade during Madame's French class.

22. I have vivid, bizarre nightmares most nights.

23. If my life were different, I would've joined the Peace Corps.

24. I don't wear my hair in ponytails because I think it accentuates my pinhead.

25. I am 25 years old, which is neither random nor interesting, but it's the number of things I just wrote.

⬥

1/1/2010

CAITLIN: Love you. Love when I see the new year. It's all just a weird time construct but I hope I see blue moon 2015!! Love you so much.

⬥

The night before Nick and I were to meet Caitlin in Boston to fly to Pittsburgh, I was alone in our house and turned on the TV. *Steel Magnolias* happened to be playing. I had never seen it, but I knew it was heart-rending and that a daughter died. At the end, I was sobbing into the sofa.

We were finally facing what we had tried for so long to prevent. Pittsburgh was her only shot.

Unlike the Boston experience, the UPMC evaluation would take place within one calendar week. We knew to expect multiple physical tests and interviews, followed by a judgment: she would or would not be accepted as a transplant candidate.

⬥

Pittsburgh. City of bridges. Cold, overcast air that smelled of burning coal. Taxis that allowed smoking. Panic building inside me until I met Dr. Joe Pilewski. Then relief replaced my qualms. He was clearly one of the exceptional doctors and spoke very plainly and eloquently about having a moral responsibility to transplant people with cepacia.

Later that first morning, at an orientation talk, a man spoke. He'd had the first single lung transplant at Pittsburgh. In 1991. Five years later, after a bout of pancreatitis that led to organ failure and three years of living on a ventilator, he had a double lung transplant. He was in a coma for two weeks. He was 110 pounds when he was released. He fell and broke his hip—and then needed a kidney transplant as well. He survived nearly two decades of terrible health. Now he was in his sixties. His FEV1—the volume of air you can force out in one second after you take a deep breath—was now 112, and he worked out hard five days a week. Loved to golf.

More proof that you just never know what's going to happen in this life. So why not be positive?

☙

October 6, 2010

9:30
In waiting room. Just sent Caitlin a text: "I am the glamorous type," and waited, watching, to see her laugh.

9:45
Now she's doing a six-minute walk test. Tech hasn't stopped her so she must be doing okay.

10:45

Last appointment of the day. Things have gone rather smoothly. A bit daunting to think of what it would entail to be here for many weeks, but thank God we can manage it, and there are people to help.

The great news was that Dr. Pilewski said that if her current baseline holds steady, she can hopefully put off transplant for two or three or maybe even five years. They're always hoping for better anti-rejection drugs to come along, which could make all the difference to outcome.

He also addressed a big fear of mine when he said that nearly everyone survives the actual operation. I did not know that. It's the first year that generally determines how well someone will do.

October 8

Home. Awake. It's 1:30 a.m. Quiet night. Sky full of stars, reflecting in the river. Imagining the reality of getting the call—the race to the airport, bag pre-packed.

But it's not now.

So no need for anxiety now.

Wednesday, October 13

Good news. Accepted, but hopefully she can get a good couple of years, maybe more, before she needs to be listed. Thank God and the universe.

Did this help me? This ability to compartmentalize, to put CF back in its box, a reconfigured one once again but a box all the same?

I think so. I can still feel the sweet relief of being able to push transplant away and let myself hope big: that maybe a miracle of science would happen and it would never have to take place. That our cat would get every one of her nine lives.

From the earliest days of her diagnosis, I had a maxim that I could easily follow as long as we weren't in crisis: *Don't ruin today worrying about tomorrow.*

I followed it now, filled with a renewed sense of expanding time. I could focus on myself for a while. I vowed to finish my novel, which I did, up on the seacoast during the final days of 2010.

From: Caitlin O'Hara
To: A childhood friend
Date: May 21, 2015
Subject: Looking back through my 20s

Well, I had pretty much been in "poor" health from age 24 and on. Except it was not so bad that I couldn't fake it and kind of live normally. But I also couldn't strike out and do something bold. It really was this constant picking and choosing of battles/fun/etc.

It is so hard to explain, but I will try. I see a lot of CF people go through the same thing. It's like you aren't sick enough to have your quality of life completely suffer. But when you have fun in the scope of "normal 20-something fun" . . . whether it's as simple as drinks after work (drinking anything, anytime basically, no matter how little), or a weekend away, or a vacation in the Caribbean, your health suffers.

So life becomes this lead-up to preparing for the hit your body will take for the fun you want to have and then the subsequent recovering from it. But that somehow feels like the only way to lead the fairly normal fun life you want to lead. And from the outside it looks like you just do what everyone else does and it's not that big a deal, but really there is a lot a lot of juggling involved, decision-making. A weekend spent partying cannot be followed up by another weekend partying without consequences. Or, if a trip is planned in the winter, during the weeks before, you might choose to stay home and not have dinner with friends, or a casual after-work drink, because you don't want to risk catching a cold and missing your trip (this happened many times to me).

You get disappointed a lot, abandoning plans you can't keep. And everyone thinks you are normal so it always feels like you are saying no to people and even though they understand that "you're tired" or whatever, it just doesn't make sense to them. Like, if I really wanted to go to a party on a Friday night, it would mean I couldn't have dinner with Allison on Thursday night. And that is hard for people to understand. Because on Thursday night there is nothing actually wrong with me and I'm not "sick."

Anyway . . . so imagine that mentality is your way of living, and then it just feels like, is it all worth it? It is all two steps forward one step back, or sometimes one step forward and two steps back, but never really going anywhere. And I don't know what I was waiting for, because I knew I wasn't getting any healthier. That kind of became obvious around age 25 . . . but it was a slow, slow decline, obviously, to now. I was also too healthy for transplant. So it's just like, this *wait*.

4

REPRIEVE,
DENIAL,
REPRIEVE

11/23/2011

CAITLIN: i felt like i was gaining weight this week even though I'm
not like eating a TON. i just got on the scale. granted i just ate
but still 110.5 wtf
MARYANNE: Kalydeco ☺
CAITLIN: so now I'm like a regular person who gets fat from eating
6 or 7 bon bons a day and marcona almonds and a chocolate
croissant and a hot chocolate and 2 eggs and a bagel with cream
cheese and salmon and raspberries and blueberries and a jumble
nut cookie?
MARYANNE: tee hee

Twenty-six years after her diagnosis, Caitlin was frequently asked to speak at CF functions and to business groups about Kalydeco, the life-changing, game-changing, gene-modifying drug she had begun to take.

Within hours of taking it for the first time, in July, she felt palpably "better." As it became part of her daily regimen of meds, she gained weight, normally a struggle. Her skin, no longer salty, stopped fading her bedding and clothing. Most remarkably, she experienced fewer lung infections and would go a year and a half without needing an IV antibiotic cleanout.

> *O for a time machine, a lifetime supply of magic blue pills delivered to babyhood!*

If Kalydeco had existed before her lung damage began, it might have been as good as a cure.

The day I sat down to write this section, by coincidence I found a list of her handwritten notes from a 2011 speech, stuffed inside a cookbook:

> *I'm 28.*
> *History of fundraising from my perspective . . .*
> *Born—life expectancy 18.*
> *0% gene had been identified*
> *few medicines*
> *"we don't know"*
> *"she could be gone by Christmas"*
> *"be around forever."*
> *This year a new drug was approved.*
> *Vertex Pharmaceuticals, VX-770, Kalydeco.*
> *Little blue pill that actually fixes the genetic defect in CF. It's*

amazing. The thing is, it only targets one mutation of the CF gene,
and only 4% of CF people have that mutation.
Luckily, me.
Lots of benefits
Unluckily, a little too late for me.
I might look completely normal, but—
You: 100% lung function.
I have 30%.

To give you an idea of how slow the process is, I started using
oxygen in 2005 to sleep and to fly. Evaluated for transplant in
2010. I'm still not considered sick enough for transplant.

Quality of life:
No stairs
No high heels
Driving everywhere.

Thirty percent of normal lung function can look, on the outside, like normal. During her nearly three-year wait for transplant, Caitlin's lung function hovered between 18 and 20 percent of normal. Yet whenever she removed her oxygen cannula from her face, she looked, with her long blond hair and young face, normal. She looked like Caitlin.

CF is a mostly invisible disease, and if I, her mother, could sometimes be fooled by it, it's not surprising that other people often just didn't quite get it.

Even now, I have to remind myself: Don't be quick to judge people. So much that we humans suffer with is invisible.

An astrological reading that I had done in 2009—for bemused fun but it was remarkably accurate—had suggested that in the next few years I was going to become deeply involved in spiritual pursuits. I had dismissed that. I'd been researching and writing my novel for too many years. I wanted to finish it, see it published, do a book tour. I wanted some worldly success.

In early 2011, I got what I had worked for: an agent, and a publishing contract with Viking Penguin.

But that same spring, I also signed up to take a Reiki class. Even as I filled out the online registration form, I honestly didn't know what was compelling me to do it. I didn't quite believe in Reiki, or even know what it really was, just that it was a form of energy work, where the practitioner held his or her hands over various parts of the client's body. I had sampled a session at a health fair, years before, and felt nothing.

But Caitlin and I had long experienced those unexpected, powerful energy exchanges. I was curious to know whether I could learn to harness that energy, control it.

I was willing to try anything that might help stave off transplant.

I enrolled in a two-day course in the Usui system of Reiki at the New England School of Acupuncture, thinking that if the class turned out to be a bunch of weirdos I would just leave. Instead, the group was made up primarily of nurses and a couple of people, like myself, who wanted to help a sick family member.

The class was serious but refreshingly low-key. It turned out that I had randomly signed up with a well-known, respected, and very down-to-earth longtime practitioner, Libby Barnett. Libby laughed a lot and did not take herself too seriously. She described how she had, rather serendipitously, come to Reiki herself.

In a Reiki class, the instructor trains the students in Reiki techniques and then "attunes" each student to various levels of "universal energy." At the end of the first course day, we all sat quietly in our chairs, eyes closed, hands clasped, heads down as Libby approached us, one by one.

After my attunement, head still bent, I opened my eyes and spread out my hands. Long beams of white, dusty-looking light extended from each fingertip.

I blinked a few times, to focus and see if the beams would disappear. I flexed my fingers and moved them out and around, out and around. The light beams moved with my fingers, clear, consistent, visible.

I told myself, *Whatever this is, it is real. It is happening.*

The beams faded after everyone had been attuned and the class resumed. No one else had experienced those beams. But they came back for my second attunement the next day, and six months later, after daily practice and weekly volunteer sessions on inpatients at Brigham and Women's Hospital, for my final master's attunement.

Ten long beams of dusty-looking white light, stretching into infinity.

It was a few months after the Reiki classes and Caitlin was living in Boston, working at the graphic design school, thriving as well as her damaged lungs could thrive on the Kalydeco drug. And I was living my own life again. Working on the edits for my forthcoming novel. Deep into researching a new one about the ambiguities of human memory. Volunteering at Brigham and Women's Hospital, where I discovered that the true gift of Reiki is closing a patient's door, turning on soft music, and providing the patient with twenty minutes of undisturbed, kind attention.

I was letting myself dare to hope for a very long reprieve from transplant. In fantasy moments, I even let myself dream of a forever reprieve. A BU researcher who lived near my brother was studying stem cells and lung tissue regeneration. I knew such science was years away, but Caitlin had plateaued at a livable baseline and stayed there for a long time. With the help of the Kalydeco, maybe she could stay at this baseline for years and then . . .

One late summer day she came home for Sunday dinner. We sat in our three chairs at our round kitchen table, windows open to let in the breeze. Our house was like the three bears' house except we called ourselves the three pigs. We had three of everything: three bathrooms, three dining chairs, three armchairs in a little alcove we called the "pig room."

On this day I had hidden a tiny rubber donkey under Caitlin's napkin—it was an old joke having to do with our favorite vacation spot, St. John, where wild donkeys roam the hills and block the roadways. The three of us were laughing about something when Henry interrupted. He needed to go out.

I walked him down the patio steps to the lawn. The grass was yellow with the setting sun and there was a soft wind off the river. I could hear the faint sounds of Caitlin and Nick talking, and a little bit of laughter. The two of them were alike—strong-willed people who didn't like to be told what to do. They'd not enjoyed a friction-free relationship but now that she was an adult, they shared an easier camaraderie and I loved hearing them laugh. Henry was scampering ahead of me, heading back up to the house, but I paused and tried to hold on to the moment, the now that was briefly so perfect.

Note Found Among Caitlin's Papers

April 27, 2012

I am grateful for:

My parents
My friends
My apartment & car
My dog
My ability to be able to go out and have fun even though I'm sick

❦

After a year of stable health thanks to Kalydeco, Caitlin traveled alone to Paris, as she had dreamed of doing for years. She saved all winter. Rented an apartment in the twelfth. Stuffed an enormous suitcase full of weeks' worth of medicine vials, syringes, nebulizer cups, nebulizer machine, and a six-pound portable oxygen concentrator.

Squeezed to one side: only the tiniest bundle of clothes and toiletries.

Why did things never seem to go completely right for her? It was as if every event in her life had to be a trial. She had done everything right. Researched. Rented a well-rated apartment with an elevator. But the elevator broke the day she arrived. She was on the sixth floor. It took twenty minutes for her to climb the stairs and then she was afraid to go out again. She emailed updates.

Ugh. Elevator still not fixed. Spoke to sort of scary housekeeper who had her feet up and just said "J'attende." And shrugged. She said it would be today though. Hard to get cabs. Regretting my location.

I coughed up blood and I feel awful bc of the no sleep and oxygen. Feel really overwhelmed by the heat and no elevator. And needing to get things. I know it will be ok but I had to say it.

It was okay in the end, and she would later say that spending those weeks in Paris, alone, was one of the best times of her life. She visited churches and museums at her own pace. From a movie theater, she sent me a photo of purple velvet walls and wrote,

I was thinking about the ends of things that I love. The end of *Anna Karenina*. The end of *Ulysses*. The end of the movie *Crimes and Misdemeanors*. It is a voice over by the (made-up) philosopher in the movie *Louis Levy*, who is based on Primo Levi . . .

She bought herself a ring, delicate and shaped like a bird with long, tapered wings.

Then I went to the Marais for a shawarma and walked around. Then I was still hungry so I went to this crepe place and had two giant crepes—1 savory—egg sunny side up, ham, raw milk gruyere, and artichoke. And then a sweet one—chocolate, pear and whipped cream. It was a nice place, a real restaurant that I had heard about— the savory ones are really "galettes" made with whole wheat buckwheat and all the other ingredients were from different dairy farms. Delicious! I took a picture of the savory one and tweeted it. I forgot to take a picture of the sweet one! Piggy.

I realized something I've loved about being here—I finally feel on par with the schedule that is suited to me, like as related to the US. I don't wake up to a million emails from everyone who has already been up for hours. I know we only feel how we let ourselves feel, BUT one of the "feelings" I was running from was a feeling of constantly being behind—even if I wasn't (or if it didn't matter). I find myself rushing in the morning always, even if I always always always get to work around 11:30–12, and it never matters, no one cares . . . there is this back of the mind feeling continuously of "you're last, you're late, you're behind." I fight it. Or it's more a constant justification like "don't feel bad Caitlin, your job is flexible, you can do what you want, who cares what people say ("early start huh?"). Here I wake up and it's 4 am at home. I have my day and people don't start contacting me until midafternoon, right around the time I start to feel great. By the time I get home to rest or whatever, whether its 7pm, or 9pm, I can do my work then, and it is still the work day. It suits me perfectly. I love not waking up to a barrage of emails. By midnight I can talk to my friends a little who are just ending their day and then I can go to bed.

Also no one here eats at 5 or 6 or even 7. They all eat at 8 or 9 or 10. I love it! And I can eat lunch at 3:30 or 4 which is so much more natural to me.

I love you!

Summer in Paris was followed by new love. It was that kind of year. On a balmy night in Portsmouth, New Hampshire, on an outing with Katie, Fate introduced Caitlin to Andrew, who was from southern Maine and walking around, in need of directions. He ended up joining them at a diner and she told me about him the next day. He was "different," she said. "Interesting."

A week later, we were about to head up to Portland, Maine, for a book reading and party for me when she said, "I think I'll drive my own car. I'm going to meet that guy for a day date, see how it goes. I'll meet up with you guys at the hotel."

Hours later I got a phone call. "Is it okay if he comes to the reading? We're having such a good time!"

It's an interesting thing to look back, later, on when you first met a person who would forever after be an important character in your life story. That night, Andrew sat in the back row at my bookstore reading and paid attention. At the party afterward, he fit in with no fuss. His manner was direct but easygoing and I detected a sense of humor, always a good thing.

The next morning, I joined Caitlin in her hotel room and she told me all about the day date in Ogunquit, the seaside town where Andrew lived. She said he was very smart and kind and that they had talked instantly and forever about "things."

"It's like he's the male version of me," she said. Then her face went a bit white. "O God, that's what that psychic told me, that I would be the female version of this guy I was going to meet."

A friend had persuaded her to talk to a psychic a few weeks earlier, and she had rolled her eyes at the psychic's assurance that a good man was about to come into her life. She hadn't been interested, hadn't been looking. "I'm taking a break from guys," she'd told the psychic.

But it turned out to be true. Andrew and Caitlin were very similar people: intelligent, even-tempered, and open-minded, and at the same time rigid about certain things, mainly morality. They both possessed strong moral compasses.

On the August day when my publisher officially launched my novel, I was scheduled to talk on one of Boston's public radio shows. It was a Thursday, the day I volunteered at the hospital. It felt important to stay grounded during this time, so I decided to stick with my schedule and go to the hospital after the interview.

As I was driving down Huntington Avenue, I heard a message that I can only describe as words in my mind, clear and firm and not my own.

You're supposed to help people into the next life.

What? I didn't want to hear that. I didn't even know what it would entail, though I know now that it meant doing what I'm doing here, right now, with these pages. Personal sharing. But back then?

No.

❦

Note Found Among Caitlin's Papers

September 12, 2012

Waiting on blood work and doctor's call. Stressed. Scared. I don't know if having another disease is something I can handle. So much time thinking about myself. Feel depleted. So much time just trying to care for myself that I have no energy left to really truly do something outside of me. Wish I could just forget about myself and throw myself into something meaningful but the mundane daily aspects of health keep me tethered to my stupid problems.

Feel desperately hopeful now that Obama will win. Biden's speech about his grandmother and courage.

Courage. That word means it all to me.

When I feel myself flailing, grasping, panicking with pain or hurt, I get a notion in my head, always, and remember that there is courage.

Courage is the answer. Because courage doesn't negate the problem, it exists within the problem. And when you realize the

answer lies in taking in the problem and living in spite of it,
with full awareness of it, you feel a new option and a new sense
of hope and life.

12/18/2012

MARYANNE: are you okay bud
CAITLIN: yea, i just feel really weird
in a bad way
MARYANNE: what can you do
CAITLIN: there isn't anything i can do really, migraines are like just
really hard to prevent.
they make no sense
just eat and drink and sleep
but i mean it might not matter
i did that all day yesterday and got the worst one
CAITLIN: my risk of stroke is significantly higher which freaks
me out
and there is this thing where you can have a stroke during
migraine with aura
i mean it's not truly harmless
MARYANNE: you are NOT going to check out of here by stroke, i
know it
CAITLIN: whatever mom, thank you
but i don't think you know everything
CAITLIN: I've always thought i was going to die of a stroke

Did I try too hard to pretend that life was normal? Did she hesitate to tell me what she knew I didn't want to hear? Something shifted in her in 2013, and my journal shows me exactly when.

In late spring, I met her at a favorite spot for lobster BLTs. She had just come from a routine CF appointment and I was helping her plan her upcoming thirtieth birthday on July 31. She and Andrew were planning a big trip to Ireland. They had booked Aer Lingus tickets to Shannon, where they would join Katie and her husband. All through their growing-up years, Katie and Caitlin had planned a someday trip to the holiday home that Katie's grandparents owned on the western peninsula of Dingle. Now it would finally happen. Then they would visit Nick's family on the eastern coast, where Nick grew up. She would get to see all her family, and was most excited to see her cousin Sinéad, who'd visited our home in the US so often, all her life, that the two cousins had developed a strong bond.

As a gift, we were giving them miles to fly home comfortably, in business class, on American Airlines.

"I've always felt like something is going to happen when I'm thirty," she said in the middle of our chat.

"Jesus," I said, "don't say things like that!" I pointed out that she hadn't needed a cleanout in more than a year, that I'd been volunteering at the Brigham for a year and a half, and it was crazy how she had never once been an inpatient during my time there. "And you're going to go on this trip you've always wanted to go on," I said. "Dingle with Katie!"

But she was pushing her salad around the plate, something bothering her.

It was the CT scan. "The tech was this guy my age and we got talking. He asked me all these questions, just out of curiosity."

She'd told him about her slow decline, about how her failing lungs were affecting her heart, how she now had frequent, frightening episodes of supraventricular tachycardia (SVT)—heart racing out of control—that landed her in the emergency room. Every few months, she found herself giving up more and more activities.

"He asked why didn't I just get a transplant and I explained that basically you have to wait until your quality of life is intolerable, then you get listed, and he said, 'Wow, so basically you're living in limbo.'

"He made me really see it, Mom. My life is limbo."

Her life was limbo, and going to Ireland would be a mistake. I sensed it then. I know it now. It's a damp country and she got sick and very stressed and she never recovered.

Still, she'd always known that having an illness meant navigating the balance between two choices: *Live like an invalid, or live.*

⋙

In October, after a 3½-week cleanout, which took place after the 2-week cleanout she did when she finally limped home from Ireland, I visited her in Boston.

She was sitting on the sofa, computer on her lap, working. Looking normal except for the oxygen cannula on her face, connected to the large oxygen concentrator that was normally by her bed, for nighttime use only.

It was the first time I'd seen her use oxygen just to exist, to sit on a sofa.

"It makes me feel better." She spoke defensively.

Panic, already simmering. Turning into denial. *This is just a blip, she will get back to her baseline. Oxygen is a good idea, anything to help her get back to her baseline.*

❦

Caitlin once wrote that she was a pathological nonplanner, that "with an illness, sometimes you stop making plans to avoid disappointment." We never planned trips far in advance. We were too afraid to jinx them, but at some point, if you wanted your choice of accommodations, you had to start booking.

In late November, Caitlin was finally back to using oxygen just for sleeping and I dared to book a January trip to our beloved island of St. John. I reserved our favorite villa, one that sat high on a hilltop, with a 180-degree view of green islands and aqua sea. I also booked "boat day," our favorite part of a vacation, a day when we popped on and off many of the British Virgin Islands.

Katie and her husband were going to come, as would Andrew. Andrew had joined us the previous year and loved the island too, waking at dawn to hike down to the ocean—even taking Caitlin along one exhilarating day when they realized she could hike *down*hill and he could piggyback her up any inclines.

A few weeks later, I planned for Katie and her mom to drive down from New Hampshire and meet us at Caitlin's apartment; then we would all attend the annual Holiday Stroll on Charles Street in Boston.

At her apartment, Caitlin opened the door and welcomed us in, looking wonderful. Normal. She had even had the energy to buy herself a live, tabletop Christmas tree and decorate it.

We all did the kind of accommodating we didn't think twice

about, taxiing the short distance from Caitlin's apartment to the far end of Charles Street so that Caitlin had to stroll only one way.

There were carol singers on the sidewalks and treats inside the holiday-lit shops. We ate salads and thin, crispy pizzas at Scampo, a favorite restaurant. I kept telling myself that life was back to normal, and I kept talking about St. John, as if I could will it into happening.

At one point Caitlin turned to me and said, "I think I'm getting a darn cold again." My heart skipped with fear but she was quick to reassure me. "It's just a cold," she said. "It's not like before."

❧

12/20/2013

MARYANNE: I hope this lack of emails for a long time means you slept well?
CAITLIN: Slept better than I did the other nights. From about 12:45–now.
I kept waking up thinking how I didn't want to wake up and deal with how sick I feel. I also caved and took beta blockers.
How are u.
MARYANNE: Still the same?
CAITLIN: Yes same. Worse? Idk. Like short of breath so badly. Walking to kitchen and sucking air.
But sometimes I feel terrible too and am not sucking air and sats are low.
Anyway it feels awful and scary. I don't think I can sit here all day thinking about it. Like I want to go out anyway.
MARYANNE: Maybe you should come home, bud.

On Christmas Day, as Katie and I talked in our hyped-up, excited way about the St. John trip, I read Caitlin's face. It was a game face. A few nights before, her SVT had been so bad she and Andrew had spent the night in the ER. I knew she was thinking that there was no way she would be able to go on vacation.

The house was full of people and cooking and Christmas music, the background buzz high with talk and laughter. After our afternoon feast, we prepared for more people later in the evening, for something we called our annual Barrel Party. Out on the brick patio, Nick filled an old barrel full of firewood. I served trays of Irish coffee in traditional glasses, with Jameson whiskey and fresh whipped cream. Everyone stood under the stars and watched the flames and laughed and talked, and Barrel Party nights were full of merriment.

Caitlin was feeling too sick to attend the Barrel Party part of the day. I was up and down the stairs, attending to the party and then back up, checking on her. She was worsening by the hour, and at one point I stood on the staircase, on that same tread where I had told myself, long ago, *It's not over.* I listened to the sounds of thirty people laughing and enjoying the holiday in the home Nick and I had made from nothing. Then I entered her room full of a *let's do this!* attitude and talk.

I would remain in desperate denial for a couple of weeks, but at one point I said to Katie, "She's either going to get better, like she always has, or we are entering a whole new place with this disease."

That January was a blur of motion, an all-day-long busy house: med preparations, cooking, breakfast, lunch, dinner, snacks. Every action infused with prayer. *Gain weight, please gain weight.* Every organic vegetable, every piece of free-range protein. *Please nourish her, please make her well.* Tap tap, meds. *Clear her lungs, make her well.*

I canceled the St. John trip, and a long-planned visit to Big Sky with my college friends.

She stayed in the guest bed for weeks. She, who never complained, admitted that she had never felt this bad, that if she could get a transplant "right this minute, I would."

I cooked all of her meals, serving them on cheery trays, with sprigs of holly or a flower in a vase. Always trying to be positive, to will a good outcome. I'd randomly put on a song like Pharrell Williams's joyous "Happy" and dance silly, in place, to make her laugh.

A home-care nurse came once a week to check her line, change the dressing, draw blood for labs in that room that was always chaotic and messy, no matter how hard I tried to keep it organized, with its bags and boxes of supplies, and dragged-in tables filled with trays spilling over with the day's syringes and vials and the Sharps container and bags stuffed with all the medical waste a cleanout generates—tubing and plastic wraps and bandages and latex gloves and gowns and her clothes strewn around, books, magazines, snacks, Clif Bars, jugs of water, electronics, chargers.

To save her breath, she would text me.

CAITLIN: I feel so sad thinking about my dead little Christmas tree
I feel like I just abandoned my apartment.
Like I'm in this weird world and I'm losing my other life

She didn't take a shower for two weeks—didn't have the breath to take off the oxygen long enough to do it—until we realized that it was possible to wear an oxygen cannula in the shower.

There was so much we didn't know.

For a month, until her lack of improvement forced her hand, she was adamant about not going into the hospital, afraid she would catch the flu or other virus that would make her even sicker and throw her off the cliff for good.

She finally capitulated. And the bittersweet part was that being in the Brigham was pleasant and easier. The hospital room contained a microwave and refrigerator so she could easily consume her own food. And extra, healthy options provided by the hospital were just a phone call away, any time of the day or night.

Good nurses, good therapists. Such all-around good medical care. A Brigham transplant doc who squeezed her hand and said, with real anguish, *I wish we could transplant you here!*

Ahmet Uluer, her pulmonologist for the past half-dozen years, whom she trusted and loved, asked again, but the official verdict from the Brigham transplant team was still a blanket *no* to ceno-cepacia patients.

Katie regularly drove down from New Hampshire and burst into the room to fix Caitlin's hair or give her massages, and there would be hours of talking and joking that felt painfully near to normal life.

We were desperate for normalcy, but there was nothing we could do except admit that the trajectory of our lives had changed. The seasons were not going to roll out ahead of us like they always had. She was going to be reevaluated for transplant, for listing this time, 551 miles away, in western Pennsylvania.

All we could do was submit to it.

And now it's another January and I stand in her bedroom, so quiet and spare now, the bed neatly made. I open the bedside drawer. Inside are some of her digestive enzymes, a couple of scrunchies, a small white notebook.

The word LIFE is printed in red on the cover. She had written on only one page, the first.

5

IT BEGINS

Hurry up and wait. The medical jet that was to take us to Pittsburgh at first light for the transplant reevaluation was routed to Florida to deal with an emergency. By the time the coordinating ambulance collected us from the Brigham, it was dark, late, and very cold.

The ambulance was bright and orderly inside, the EMTs polite and professional. We moved through the streets of Boston, then down Route 9 and up Route 128 and finally turned onto Hanscom Field, a small, public-use airfield.

We waited in the ambulance. Outside, nothing stirred.

It was close to midnight when the plane appeared, taxiing in much tinier than I expected—the kind of Cessna you can't stand up in.

The crew—two pilots and a nurse—swiftly went into action. They were cordial but all business, bundling Caitlin into the rear of the plane with oxygen and monitors. Then they motioned me to get in.

After the bright, organized ambulance, the interior of that

cramped tin can, cluttered and dark, filled me with panic. I thought, *You can't get into that thing*.

But I had to get into that thing. They stuffed me into a pop-up seat behind the pilot and immediately we were off, our bodies hurtling through the dark night, the engine noise deafening, conversation impossible.

I could see the moon through the cockpit window. It was a waxing crescent moon.

I thought about how we were flying on faith. We did not know what would happen. I didn't even know if we would stay in Pittsburgh until she was transplanted, but Dr. Uluer seemed to think we might. How long would that be? Once you needed surgery, you wanted it right away, of course. But she wasn't even listed yet. Four years had passed since her evaluation. Her condition had to be reassessed. All was uncertain.

❧

Two a.m. disorientation. Deserted streets, the hospital sitting high on the steep incline I remembered was nicknamed Cardiac Hill. Wheeling through silent halls to what someone called the lung floor. An old-fashioned, never-updated, 1960s kind of hospital room.

Caitlin sat within the confines of the bed while I put on latex gloves and went to work wiping down every surface, as I always did, with heavy-duty disinfecting wipes. Toilet handles, light switches, doorknobs. Then she unpacked her toiletries and went into the bathroom to wash up.

I looked out the window. Nothing to see but another dark building.

Staff came in and out. It always took a while to get meds ordered.

Someone said that since it was the middle of the night, they probably would not do the intake until morning.

Okay. Fine. We turned out the lights. Caitlin fell asleep. I settled into an awkward reclining chair.

At 3:00 a.m., maybe four, sudden overhead light woke us. A resident. "I'm here to do your intake," she said.

More fitful sleep, then, very early—6:00 a.m.?—a respiratory therapist knocked. He said he was there to do what he called Caitlin's breathing treatment.

I whispered so she wouldn't wake up. "You mean her inhaled ceftaz?"

"Yes."

"Oh, she never does it this early."

But she was awake now, too, and waving him away. "I don't do that now. I can't do it until after I've been awake for a while."

He said it was required that he stay and observe her while she did it.

She laughed at that and explained that the treatment didn't do her any good unless she had been up and moving awhile.

Another knock. "Dietary!"

A beige hospital tray containing gelatinous eggs, white toast, a weight-gain shake in a tiny carton that listed corn syrup as the primary ingredient.

"I can't eat that," she said. "It's not even healthy."

In the hospital settings Caitlin had known, CF patients like her were known to be competent, savvy. They'd taken care of themselves their whole lives. As inpatients, they were generally free to follow their own schedules.

Now a nurse entered the room. He insisted that he needed to record her taking her digestive enzymes with the breakfast she told him she had no intention of eating.

Caitlin, beloved all her life by her medical teams in Boston, was coming across as difficult.

I was getting a little panicky. Were we in the right place?

We had to be, when it was the only place.

I wheeled my bag along the sidewalk to a tall, pale brick structure located among other UPMC and University of Pittsburgh buildings. A staff member had given me information about Family House, which offered a homelike setting to families of patients. I rang the bell and took an elevator up to the reception desk, where a woman asked how she could help, and smiled at me with such kindness that I lost my ability to speak. I was suddenly choking with grief and tried to compose myself, wipe my eyes.

"It happens all the time," she said.

I was grateful she was so kind. And I was in luck. There was a room available.

She showed me around: a large double kitchen, laundry room, television corners, a couple of spacious sitting areas. There were two floors below, she said, which housed the bedrooms. She gave me the key for mine.

I rolled my bag down to my room and unlocked the door. A clean set of folded sheets sat at the end of the bed. There was a bureau and a tall dresser with a television on top of it. A bathroom. Windows that faced the hospital compound.

I gazed out the window, picturing Caitlin inside her room. I wondered how she was faring. I thought about Henry and how I wished I could hold him and kiss his little golf ball head, all of us home, none of this happening.

But when I got back to the hospital, Caitlin reported that

things were better. Betsy, a CF nurse practitioner on the floor, was very good, she said, and had let the staff know that Caitlin had made it this far in life because of how well she had taken care of herself.

It turned out that for as many lung transplants that they do in Pittsburgh, few recipients are young CF patients like Caitlin. They are generally older people who have only recently had to live with medical issues, and compliance can be a problem.

I was in the Family House kitchen, preparing a dinner plate for Caitlin. Twice a day, a housekeeping team scoured the place, but I was still paranoid. I wiped down everything communal with disinfectant wipes and kept her items on clean paper towels.

An older woman wearing oxygen rolled in in a wheelchair. She began to assemble a sandwich and tell me all about herself. She was waiting for a lung transplant, too. At first she and her husband had waited at home, with a free Angel Flight on standby, because technically they could get to Pittsburgh within the four-hour window required by the transplant team. She had been listed for only a few weeks when she got the call. "But it was a dry run," she said. Since they had used up their Angel Flight credit and figured it would likely be no time until she got another call, they had decided it made economic sense to relocate to Pittsburgh to wait.

Now she had been waiting nearly a year. I could see that she was normally a cheerful, nice person, but the experience had made her bitter. She alluded to other people being taken to transplant "out of turn."

I didn't know what she was talking about. I was focused on one fact: that she had been waiting a year.

"I cannot imagine being here for a year," I said.

"Oh, one woman was here from Italy. She waited two years!"

Two years. I looked down at the broccoli I was buttering to hide my eyes as they filled.

"Oh, but she got her transplant," she said. "She got it and eventually went home."

There were so many difficult stories. We were just one of them.

I look at our gchats from those March days when she was in her hospital bed and I was back in my room at Family House. Our correspondence was fraught with anxiety about the reevaluation—what if something came up that would be a deal breaker for listing her?

At one o'clock one night, she was worried about her right foot. *It's swollen and I've been extra breathless all night.*

But we also talked about making sure we got our taxes done, and she sent me a half-dozen links to outfits she liked on Shopbop. She used her iPad to binge-watch *House of Cards.* I texted her some Kristin Wiig impersonations I was watching on YouTube. *Oh, Barbie!*

Jess sent photos from Nanyuki, Kenya, where she was helping to organize a program that would get homeless kids off the street and back into school. The photos were of children and zebras and sunrises she said were like nowhere else on Earth. Jess can present as stereotypically "American"—natural blond hair, wide blue eyes, a voice with a bit of vocal fry. Yet Africa had called to her heart for years, ever since she first visited as an eighteen-year-old and knew she'd found her soul's home.

Caitlin was afraid that Jess would end up living permanently in a place she feared she could never visit. She forwarded the pictures

to me with hopeful commentary: *Maybe I can go after transplant.*
Meg went to China after her transplant.

You'll be able to do anything! I replied. But Kenya and China
seemed impossibly far away when even home seemed like a lost
place. Nick and Andrew were flying in in a few days but I kept getting weepy about Henry. I worried that he was bereft without me.

CAITLIN: Mom. He's still getting excited for his food and wagging
his tail. Like he's not depressed.
MARYANNE: Ok. Right. I guess I'll get some sleep. Xoxo
CAITLIN: love you
MARYANNE: love you bud. pup
CAITLIN: pupologist

Late one night I walked into the Family House kitchen. Two young
women were talking. One of them said, "Good evening" in a manner I recognized.

"You're West Indian?"

"How do you know?"

From our many St. John trips, I knew that West Indians always
began conversations with a formal *Good morning, Good day,* or *Good*
evening.

She was Teppany, so composed and self-assured that she
seemed older than her age, which I put at early thirties. Her husband, Kwesi, had had a lung transplant a month before. He didn't
have CF but something that presented like CF and was treated
like CF. In their native Trinidad and Tobago, there was no help for
him. No lung transplant opportunity. So this young woman raised
a half million dollars to pay for the portion of the surgery that their

country's medical system would not cover. They flew to Pittsburgh with two portable oxygen machines fed into one spliced nasal cannula and landed with half an hour left on the battery.

Teppany talked about UNOS scoring and how unfair it could be.

UNOS (United Network for Organ Sharing) is the private, nonprofit organization that manages the United States's organ allocation system. A transplant candidate's Lung Allocation Score (LAS) is primarily based on oxygen needs. The higher your oxygen needs, the higher your LAS score, and the likelier that you will be called.

The score doesn't strongly take into account other medical issues, such as Caitlin's increasingly severe pulmonary hypertension, caused, of course, by her failing lungs. It doesn't acknowledge that people like her purposefully keep their oxygen flow at a lower setting—say, two liters instead of four—so as not to bump oxygen saturation levels too high. Too much oxygen in the blood in a body that can't process it normally results in dangerously high CO_2.

But that was why it was good to be here in Pittsburgh, as opposed to waiting at home, Teppany said, because then you could be a "backup."

Meaning?

If lungs became available for someone, another patient was usually notified that they might be a backup, she said, in the event that the donor lungs proved to be unsuitable for the first person. They couldn't take the chance that donor organs would go to waste.

That was how Kwesi got his transplant, she said. He was allowed to be a backup because his score had not adequately reflected how critical his need had been.

Backups. This was good news.

Caitlin's overall condition had improved in just the past ten days. She had completed the reevaluation procedures, and we were basically waiting, waiting, waiting, sick with nerves, for confirmation that she would be listed.

We were in her room talking when Dr. Pilewski came in to say, Yes, the team accepts you, except he didn't say that. He talked of other things while we sat there filled with dread. He finally said, "Soo . . . there are no deal breakers. The left lung will be hard to remove, but the surgeons like a challenge, and as for the cepacia, we're not going to bring you down here and then tell you we won't transplant you 'cause of that."

So, okay. The team had accepted her. But she could not yet be listed. There were still a number of minor but necessary tests that needed to be done for final listing. And we could do those in Boston.

He was sending her home?

He advised it. Once she was listed and had a score, and that would still be a few weeks away, he could assess her likelihood of being called to transplant.

But he wasn't optimistic about that likelihood being anytime soon. He pointed out that she was petite, with O+ blood.

"Basically," he said, "you have a lot of company."

In other words, a lot of competition. Many people waiting for small, O+ lungs.

⁂

9LivesNotes Post: 4/24/2014

Caitlin: "Listed"

Caitlin here. I wasn't planning on writing on this blog but why not? "I'm not a blog person," I said. Well . . . who is? Who cares?

Why spend any time proclaiming what you are or are not, and what you don't like? There is value in that kind of thing, I know, for humor . . . but right now all I can think about is everyone I love and everything I want to do. I am so grateful for all my friends and family, for Andrew, and for my parents who continue to do anything they can for me.

So . . . I got listed today! I got my "score" which is 44. 44.2196 actually. It is a higher score than anyone expected—everyone thought I'd be somewhere in the 30's. 70's is about the highest usually. It is based on how sick you are, and you technically want it to be higher so you can get transplanted sooner. It still doesn't mean much though, and I could get called at any time, or I could wait; there is really no way to know. When there are lungs available, the calls are initially made based only on height/size and blood type. If those match up then the score comes into play, and the sickest person gets the call, and so on and so forth. That is a very simplified way of describing it. For lungs it is not a matter of having a set number in line and just waiting. Your score can change too, if you get sicker, to increase your odds of getting a transplant sooner. (All of this came in to play around 2005 when the regular wait list method wasn't working for lungs anymore.) After getting the call, I could go to Pitt and it could still be a false alarm. This happens a lot. Once they get to see the lungs in person they may decide that they aren't a good enough fit, and I come home to wait again.

I read something today somewhere, something that described transplant and waiting. I don't even know where I read it, 1 out of the 100 things I can get carried away clicking and reading. It said, "The ride of the wait is like a Six Flags Roller Coaster. Attitude will get you through most of the tough times. Believe in yourself and your inner strength to survive and NEVER give up."

Believe me, these words aren't complex, I know, but they jumped out of the page, a simple emphasis at the end of paragraphs of dry informative material. No amount of rational thinking in the world can do for you what this basic instruction can, whoever wrote this knew that, and got right down to the heart of the matter. There is no escaping that this is a risk, and we are all taking the leap—the surgeons, my family, me. And all of it manifests because someone else has to die. There is something inescapably raw about it. And at the core of it, once you have educated yourself, tried your best, and hoped the science will all work out, all you can really count on is . . . never giving up.

6

———

THIS IS NOT FOREVER

We expected to wait so it wasn't that bad in the beginning. But now I look back and feel sorry for us, for our hopefulness, for what even seems, now, to have been our naïveté.

The way I wouldn't go anywhere without a packed bag, ready to bolt.

How nervous I felt, falling asleep each night, imagining the charged fear of a 2:00 a.m. call.

We were nervous in the daytime, too. One day, Caitlin was driving and her phone rang, area code 412: Pittsburgh.

Her hands shook so hard she had to pull over to answer.

It was just a routine confirmation of an appointment that was weeks away.

Being tied to "four hours to get to Pittsburgh" meant depending on a medical air transport service, and there are surprisingly few medflight services out there, especially in Boston. Most people aren't flying *out of* Boston for medical care.

Because you cannot be guaranteed that when you need a

medflight, there will be one available to you, you have to set up a few to have on call. Then hope that luck will be with you.

❦

5/07/2014

CAITLIN: This is what has been bothering me most about our argument the other night. We need to make this time as ok and as enjoyable as possible. Who knows what's going to happen once I get that call. I don't want to live this time as if "this sucks" or "this time is really crappy and stressful." I just can't do it and I don't think it's true or smart or good for our hearts. I feel like this is your underlying sentiment despite that your brain tells you to "appreciate what we have." The truth is is that this could be it. As hard as that is to say, once I get the call I'm going into a hugely risky surgery. There aren't any guarantees. So this isn't just a time to get through—it's a time to try to be happy and make something worthwhile of it.

Everything from the bottom up here is unknown—someone has to die for me to get a transplant, so it doesn't get any more unknown or unplanned than that. The only option is to go with the flow as best we can and that means basically, assessing everything as it comes, and dealing with things but letting them go just as quickly. That includes like stress and freak-outs and fights. There's no way to avoid them so just deal with them.

This isn't a sad time we should be waiting for to be over. It will be over soon enough and you could be wishing we were back here. Or we could be glad we never have to go back here. The

point is we don't know, we can't know, and I don't want to live
like I'm just trying to get through it, when this is still my life.
I love you.

MARYANNE: I love you.

It is interesting that while you were writing that, I was making
coffee and thinking about how I needed to tell you that I feel
shame when you have to talk to me like that. You do a very good
job of taking the high road, and restraining yourself from fighting
and all that. Sorry.

CAITLIN: Ok! Be happy.

Don't feel shame. It's normal that all this will have come up. I
love you.

❧

Those first months, I collected CF/lung transplant happy-ending
stories.

John—A CF man I spoke to by phone. He told me how he had
been hospitalized and "pretty much dead," thirty years old, when
he got an eleventh-hour transplant—and this was back when transplants were still a new thing. He was now in his forties. Had married, had kids. Traveled extensively for work. I copied his Facebook
cover picture to my photo library to look at for reassurance. He
was any normal-looking, smiling, middle-aged man, photographed
with his wife and four kids.

Meg—A Boston Children's Hospital CF patient whom Caitlin
befriended over emails. Years earlier, her lungs had been ravaged
by a cepacia bug similar to the one that would keep Caitlin from
getting transplanted anywhere but Pittsburgh, but Meg was one of
the last of those cepacia patients to be transplanted in Boston. She

had a stroke during surgery, spent a month in a coma. Seven years later, she was doing so well, and was so accustomed to her antirejection therapies, that she would tell Caitlin that she didn't feel like she had CF, or *anything*, really, anymore.

Renu—Another young woman with CF, a few years younger than Caitlin, also befriended over emails. Renu waited nine long months for her transplant, during which time her need for maternal comfort was so great that she often asked her mother to sleep with her. Now she was living independently again and posted photos of herself running on the beach. She was back at Smith College, finally able to finish her degree.

Jessica—Yet another CF email friend who had waited more than a year as well, and had experienced one dry run before her successful surgery. Now she was in Key West, on a boat with her boyfriend.

I kept these stories close to my heart and shared them with friends. I meditated on them in the night when anxieties visited. I balled them up and made a fist with them. Caitlin was going to be one of these stories, too.

We humans need purpose in our lives. Look for happiness and it's hard to find. Find purpose and happiness is usually its sidekick, humming alongside.

For Nick, Andrew, and me, our common purpose was to help Caitlin stay stable and as healthy as possible for surgery.

I lived with her in her apartment during the week. On weekends, Andrew stayed over and did the cooking, cleaning, and medical help. Nick took on all the work projects his company could handle.

In July I realized I had gone six months without writing a word, and that exacerbated my general lifelong fretting about *What was I doing with my life?*, so I started a routine. I would set a timer and write for thirty minutes a day, no matter what.

It's impressive what a person can do with thirty focused minutes. Another lesson it took me a long time to learn: if something is important to you, carve out the time for it.

Caitlin spent the summer trying to occupy herself. She bought new drawing pencils and sketched birds. She taught herself to needle-felt and created small, charming animal sculptures from soft clouds of finely carded wool. She and Andrew studied for the LSAT, not because they especially wanted to go to law school but because her brain needed activity and a sense of *future*—and law school might one day appeal.

I would like to have that summer back. Let her relive it with the freedom that would have come from knowing the call to transplant was not coming.

She might have gone to Maine, to Andrew's home again. And to her beloved Martha's Vineyard, or anywhere, really, that was no more than an hour from an airport.

She didn't dare attend Katie's baby shower—the baby to whom she would be godmother—in New Hampshire. She was Kenley's maid of honor and organized an entire bachelorette weekend in the New Hampshire lakes region. The group posted photos on Instagram, and when they tagged Caitlin in them, people who didn't really know all of her details assumed she was there. It was always hard for outsiders to grasp exactly what she was going through, how she was living.

At the very last minute—the day of, to be exact—she decided to chance it and attend Kenley's wedding in Providence. Kenley was not expecting her maid of honor, and Caitlin's quiet presence, in a pew up front, was a great gift. During the reception, she cranked up her oxygen flow and used an entire tank to deliver an emotional, funny, and poignant speech. There is a snippet of video of the moment she finished. She is turning to Kenley with a beautiful smile and you can read her lips: *I love you.*

⁂

In September we had to travel to Pittsburgh for her required six-month checkup.

We had hoped that she would have been transplanted by then and we wouldn't have to make a decision about moving. But no call had come and our long New England winter was approaching. It didn't seem to make sense to stay in Boston. If the call came during bad weather, it would be impossible to get to western Pennsylvania.

Also, if she was in Pittsburgh, she could be a backup.

We planned for three nights in Pittsburgh and decided that we would find an apartment while we were there, and move by the end of the year.

We notified the medflight companies that we would be on the road, if by chance the call came while we were driving.

Four hours out of Pittsburgh, I could feel myself visibly relax. As we approached the city limits, I quietly turned on the audio system. I had secretly set it up to play the theme song from our old family favorite movie, *Groundhog Day.* The silly melody began to tinkle through the speakers, giving us all a good laugh.

Now, I thought. *Let it happen now.*

⁂

There wasn't a whole lot of rental housing that worked for us in Pittsburgh, but some friends in Boston had connections with an apartment complex in the city. An apartment was becoming available. Small but new, in a convenient downtown location, and best of all, pet-friendly. We took it with a six-month lease, to start in December.

Then we saw Dr. Pilewski.

He advised us not to move, that he didn't think she would be called anytime soon.

Caitlin pointed out that she wanted to be able to be a backup.

He pointed out that backups were rare, that a second candidate was occasionally notified to be on standby *only* if there was some concern that donor lungs might not be suitable for the intended recipient. He reminded us that all transplant teams were obligated by UNOS to follow a strict allocation sequence, thus precluding them from deciding for themselves that a patient lower on the list had more urgent need and should receive organs before a patient with a higher allocation score.

Nick and Caitlin and I looked at each other. We had just chosen the apartment, signed the lease. And going back to the stress of waiting in Boston, where her condition would undoubtedly worsen, through a long and potentially brutal winter, frightened us.

An hour later, Caitlin's transplant coordinator pointed out that local donors would always go to a local recipient, and encouraged us to make the move. "I feel better when my patients are here," she said.

Besides, in December, she would have been listed for eight months. Surely it was getting to be time for that call to come. We decided we would make the move at Christmas.

⁂

When you're desperate and you hear about a psychic who is supposedly truly gifted, you approach with a little curiosity and a lot of self-protection. If she's wrong, well, it's all just hooey. If she's right, you add it to your little arsenal of hope.

In December, right before we left for Pittsburgh, we were at a social club holiday party. I wanted to go because I knew that a psychic named Alicia would be there. She had worked an earlier summer party and we'd all been a bit blown away by her spot-on readings.

At the previous event, I noticed that Alicia seemed to tire quickly, even grow disinterested, so I got in line as soon as I arrived so I could go first. I readied the recording app on my phone and waited.

When I sat down, I said that we had a serious thing going on in our life and that I had a specific question. I briefly explained that my daughter was waiting for a lung transplant, and that I had been caring for her, and that we were moving to Pennsylvania in a week to wait for the surgery. She asked my birthday and then shuffled and seemed to speak to a deck of tarot cards. Then she asked for Caitlin's name and birthday.

She had me select six cards and then she set them out in front of her. The second one was THE LOVERS, and she tipped her head to look at me with some surprise. "Oh, she's married? Or in a serious relationship?"

"Yes, a serious relationship."

"Well, it's more than he ever expected but he's up for it and ready. He's a stand-up guy."

"He is."

The rest of the cards I had chosen showed worry for me, she said. "Not for any particular reason other than you're the mother and can't help but worry."

Then she started picking cards herself, and said, with confusion, "Wait . . . so you don't know when this is going to happen?"

"No, it's a double lung transplant. Basically, it's waiting for an organ donor . . ."

"Oh . . . I see. Right, so as for when this is going to happen, I'm not seeing it happening really soon. I'm seeing the number four. I don't know if that's four weeks or four months or what it means."

She looked at me and shrugged. "But it's still cold. Maybe toward the end of winter?"

The cars were packed. The Pittsburgh apartment was waiting. The reading was probably silly and meaningless, but it wasn't what I wanted to hear.

Oh, those first months in Pittsburgh. The anguish and uncertainty as we left Boston, everything packed into a rented, oversize SUV, Caitlin's fear as we closed the door on her apartment, the way she gripped my arm and looked from me to Andrew to Henry and back to me, her eyes round with panic. "What if I never see it again?"

"You will," I insisted, hiding my own anxiety. "You will be back! This is going to be a good thing."

We had a plan. I would stay in Pittsburgh full-time. Nick would fly out from Boston every two weeks for long weekends. And Andrew, who had been farming in Maine before winter set in, would stay with us for longer stretches, and go back, each month, to maintain his house and oversee his tenants.

We arrived a week before Christmas.

Nick had driven my car one day ahead of us so that he could set up our rental furniture, make the beds, and start to unpack. When we finally arrived, close to midnight, my eyes filled at the sight of the apartment, already cozy thanks to his efforts. He'd bought a little Christmas tree and hung strings of twinkling lights. He had votives burning and a soft blanket for Caitlin folded on the sofa.

Our place was in the heart of downtown, and downtown looked festive, with a European holiday market in the square; a skating rink; and a magical, airy public atrium filled with gingerbread houses and miniature trains.

A few days after Christmas, my sister and brother-in-law and niece visited from Maine, bearing boxes of lobsters and steamers.

Then the holidays were over. Nick and Andrew flew home with plans to return in two weeks.

January, February. *Cold. Gray. And it will last you the rest of your life.*

I could go into a litany of early complaints. That smokers were everywhere, shockingly so. That the roads were terrible to drive on and no one seemed to know how to merge onto a highway. I thought I was imagining that I was being harassed in my car with its Massachusetts plates, but it turned out, I was. Cut off, given the finger. They hated the Patriots, and when I finally put a Steelers sticker on the back of my car, the harassment stopped.

But the truth is, Pittsburgh was very very good to us. We arrived in that city knowing no one, but people were constantly offering to help us—with anything and everything—and they actually meant it. Friends of a Boston friend's husband, Ken and Sara, offered to stock our refrigerator and frequently invited us to dinners and to social events in their close and welcoming Squirrel Hill community. We couldn't do much—Caitlin was mostly housebound—and they understood yet continued to invite, to include, to remind us we weren't alone.

Jane, a writer introduced to me by Kim, another writer who only knew me by my writing and thought Jane and I would hit it off, became one of those people you meet and immediately know is a life friend. Because of writing, of art, the human need to connect.

And a friend from home connected us with some friends of his from Florida, a retired couple whose primary residence was Pittsburgh. The Cindriches invited us to a big Sunday family dinner and treated us, immediately, as if we had always been a part of their clan.

Caitlin and I were mostly companions again. Doing puzzles. Bingeing on Netflix. Going to museums or movies on once-a-week outings when she felt up for it—although she generally did not.

Her normal daily schedule consisted of multiple medicine inhalations and lots of chest physical therapy. We were back to watching old *I Love Lucy* reruns during chest PT, the way we had done during her growing-up years. She did her cardio rehab exercises— sometimes upstairs in the building's gym, at other times in the apartment with a personal leg-cycling machine and two-pound weights and *oh, the way she would close her eyes and force out a hundred arm circles, her oxygen turned all the way up*—and ate and ate and ate some more, weight gain a daily Sisyphean effort.

We put out constant little fires—most having to do with her heart, and some so frightening that during one bad stretch when Andrew was in Maine she begged me to sleep by her side.

As I write all that, I think of how she wouldn't like it. She didn't like to call attention to her troubles. She didn't complain. Her friends tell me that her first question during this time, always, was *How are you?*

There was news out of Boston. Whisperings we'd been hearing, that the administration of Children's Hospital had decided to build a new NICU and, to do it, would raze the renowned, beloved Prouty Garden, were true. We hadn't really believed it could happen. What about that plaque at the entrance to the garden, the one that proclaimed that the garden would "exist at Children's Hospital as long as there are patients, families, and staff to enjoy it"?

When word about the project had first reached hospital workers, months before, a chaplain had begun a protest campaign to point out that there were other options. But the administration had moved forward with its plans. Now Anne Gamble, a longtime hospital volunteer and wife of former cardiac surgeon Walter Gamble, had taken over the protest.

Caitlin was dismayed and could see that Anne needed help from someone like herself, digitally savvy and familiar with social media, but—getting involved in the fight, at this late date, from afar, combined with her all-day/everyday grind of self-care, overwhelmed her.

But then one day we went to see *Selma*. She came home with fire inside and contacted Dr. Elaine Meyer, the director of the Institute for Professionalism and Ethical Practices at Boston Children's Hospital, who deeply understood the importance of the garden and was trying to fight the project. The next day she spoke with Thomas Farragher, a *Boston Globe* columnist and editor who had shared the 2003 Pulitzer Prize for public service for the *Globe* Spotlight Team's coverage of the clergy sexual abuse crisis. Tom had previously included Caitlin in a column about the wonders of the Vertex Kalydeco drug, and now he wrote a column that brought much-needed public awareness to the garden's plight.

With new resolve, Anne, Elaine, and Caitlin reinvigorated The Friends of Prouty Garden, determined to save the sacred healing space. When Shelley, a young mother of a toddler who'd been born critically ill, came on board, Caitlin warned her what the group was up against: *Staff feel VERY reluctant to speak up*, she wrote. *There is a lot of subtle intimidation surrounding it. And people are not just paranoid. I love Children's, but the doctors and nurses are what I love about it. I have gone back and forth, making sure to always ask myself if I really am doing the right thing by standing up for this—and I do believe that I am. The new building will house a new NICU, yet we have NICU nurses fighting with us to save it. Same with oncology—they will benefit from the new building, yet we have oncology doctors speaking up, and one of our group, Gus, had a son die of leukemia. The hospital is just a business to the administration, and for the few who feel inclined and strong enough to stand up to them, I think it's important that we do that.*

To her Facebook community she wrote, *I feel like I have to save this garden, if I have to drag my oxygen tank in and hit someone on the head with it. It represents so much about what patients need versus what they get . . . the benefit of a natural space, a real space, outdoors. So much of the beauty of it too is that it is old fashioned, and imperfectly beautiful. Not a modern rooftop new space like lots of hospitals have. I walked here for the first time after my surgery when I was 11, the only outdoor space I saw for months. I go here every time I am at the Brigham lately. Perhaps I can never impart accurately what it means to me, what it means to someone when you are in a hospital for a long time. It just represents . . . something ELSE.*

February 2, 2015, fell on a Monday, which meant that many Groundhog Day festivities would be taking place over the weekend in Punxsutawney.

Our family favorite movie was now part of our lives in a way we could never have expected. We rewatched the movie and realized that when the opening credits panned over the city, most of the skyline was still the same, twenty-odd years later. Most hilariously surreal to us: we could clearly see the apartment where we were now living.

Punxsutawney was an hour and forty-five minutes away, a drive that would be hard on Caitlin but she wanted to do it. And, we reasoned, when would we ever be here on Groundhog Day again?

She and I drove there on a Saturday and visited Gobbler's Knob and walked around the town common and bought a wooden, top-hatted groundhog from a chainsaw artist because . . . how could we not?

02/18/2015

CAITLIN: Most days I don't feel too down but you know when you just suddenly have a moment where you feel so completely left out of life? Believe it or not I don't truly feel the pain of that much lately.

But right now I suddenly do. Andrew is up in Maine, out having fun with his friends. Carly texted me she ran into Nick in Las Vegas. Jess is in San Francisco. None of these things individually bother me, but altogether combined with everyone else I know and love just spread out doing things . . . they feel very far away. And time passes and you become so far from people's everyday life.

I had been so determined that transplant would happen quickly that I'd insisted we bring the bare minimum, going so far as to pack only one saucepan and one skillet. But the bare minimum had still resulted in two stuffed vehicles and multiple trips to Bed Bath & Beyond to buy what we realized we needed after all. There weren't enough cupboards and closets to store our clothes and food and medical supplies so we stored clothes and groceries inside boxes and suitcases. Our tiny digs grew cluttered. When Nick and Andrew were in residence, I would sometimes look up from my work and see that all four of us were wearing earbuds, everyone trying to carve out some private, quiet space.

It is temporary, I always told myself. We could survive anything for a couple of months. Friends and family helped: they visited and sent puzzles and Florida grapefruit and books and fixings for rum punch to remind us that St. John waited for us. My Boston book club even flew down for an overnight.

But every week I searched online for something more homelike and pet-friendly in the downtown area that worked for us.

No luck, but I had a secret, desperate hope that the psychic's "cold four" meant April. In April Caitlin would have been waiting a year—surely her time had to be coming. A surgery in April meant we could conceivably be on our way home by the time her recovery ended and our six-month lease expired at the end of May.

⁂

As a kid, I had wanted to travel and see every inch of the planet. Growing up in Ireland, Nick had been the same. It so took our families by surprise when we decided to marry that both mothers laughed and thought we were joking.

All of that is to say that the restrictions on me during the forced wait in Pittsburgh scared me. The lack of freedom felt like claustrophobia, like being straitjacketed. I page through my journal from those first months and they are the record of a scattered and scrambling mind: *The mind-numbing treadmill of repetitive chores. Write about what is truly important. Let the rest fall away. Hard to believe we are still waiting. Uncertainty is so hard to live with. So what is it like for people who have no one to talk to? Even though I have many who care and listen and understand, I still feel like I temper myself, aware of being on the other side, a little bit of a burden. Such an alone feeling. I don't know why we exist, why we are alive, why it's all such an intricate and marvelous set of checks and balances, this earthly life of ours. Each day waiting is another day closer, right? Car needs service, Henry to vet. Dentist. All the little things that are hard to do, away from home. It's going on so long! She's so ready. The fear that it will never happen. I'd give my life for hers, say "done" if she miraculously could have okay lungs and live a normal life. Last night I dreamed I'd been chosen to take part in some overnight, quick-ish trip to—the Mideast?—another planet? And I got back and could not remember a single detail of the journey.*

I began to use my imagination in ways I hadn't since I was a self-protecting child. I would put on electronic music as I cooked and pretend I was in Miami. Across the river from our apartment, a road snaked its way up to Mount Washington, and for the five or six seconds it took to travel a particular hairpin turn, I would exclaim, *Look, we're on St. John!* When I strolled the embankment on the Allegheny, down at the meeting of Pittsburgh's three rivers, I squinted and made horse blinders of my hands and told myself I was on the Seine. When a nearby church belfry tolled its bells for a full minute every hour, the chimes were Venice for sixty precious seconds.

April came and went. No "call to transplant," only pressure on us to decide regarding the extension of our lease. There had been a vague thought that if she hadn't been transplanted, we would go home and wait out the summer in Boston, but the reality of what that would entail overwhelmed me.

Then her health made the decision for us. In May she began experiencing lung pain, and one night her heart went into a 180-beats-per-minute state that wouldn't abate. A trip to the ER ended up in an admission as her team put her on IV antibiotics and worked to adjust her beta-blocker dose.

The lung pain became so bad she couldn't sleep. Her doctors discovered that a fungus was newly growing in her lung. Had she been transplanted before its discovery and treatment, it would have put her new lungs at much greater risk.

So. A positive.

You take positivity wherever you find it.

We were about to sign the extension on our lease, but first I did one last, desperate search for something else. This time something came up. It was almost too nice: brand new to the rental market, in a building that was mostly owner-occupied, but the deal breaker was that it required a year's lease.

I couldn't bring myself to admit that we might not be well settled at home in a year, all of this behind us. Still, I wheeled Caitlin two streets over to look at it.

The unit was modern and spacious, fifteen stories up, with big,

clear windows that overlooked the city on one side and the Monon-
gahela River on the other. Beautifully furnished, and comfortably
so, with soft white upholstery and good beds. In what seemed a
meaningful coincidence, the real estate agent's daughter had had
a heart transplant more than twenty years before and was now a
healthy, working artist.

I loved it but told myself no. The year's lease was non-negotiable
and the reality was that she could be called any day. In two or three
months, we could well be home.

But that night, wide awake in my hard rental bed in the room
with no windows, I let myself admit that we were now more than
a year into this temporary situation that had proved to be anything
but. These months were our life, and Caitlin needed comfort now
more than ever. I called Nick to discuss it, and he didn't hesitate.

I shudder now to think about how different that final year and
a half would have been if we hadn't moved. It was pretty much the
best thing we did. My sister flew in and for one week helped me
box up everything.

Seeing just how much packing and lugging it took to make the
small move from one apartment to another gave me visceral proof
of how hard it would have been to return to Boston for the summer. I wrote in my journal, *We're here and it's more of a relief than I
realized. So luxurious to be able to put things into cupboards and closets.
And best of all, Caitlin is comfortable!*

She could easily navigate the smooth floor space with her oxygen machine. The furniture and beds were of good quality and did
not make her bones ache. Sunshine filled these rooms.

It felt like a hotel, it felt like luxury. It had a small balcony and
I immediately decorated it with a potted tree, flowers, and herbs.

It felt like vacation.

We shared the fifteenth floor with only one neighbor, and when we met them, the coincidence of their identity seemed ridiculously fated. Ralph and Mary were part of the family that had invited us to Sunday dinner when we first arrived. The people who had treated us like their own.

Now Ralph and Mary were family, too.

❧

9LivesNotes Post: Mother's Day 2015

Caitlin: "Mostly Companion"

Caitlin here.

At some point when I was little, my mom and I started referring to one another as our "mostly companion." It probably grew out of the time I was having surgery when I was 11, and was in the hospital a lot. We would get overly tired, stressed, and . . . really silly. We were absurdly often at our funniest when things were worst. I guess that is common for people in trying health situations, and it's a nice silver lining. The other day, in the hospital while I tried to eat lunch, my mom put on quite a show of impressions and we were laughing so hard. The game was to do one small word, look or movement from a movie . . . not a whole line. Her imitation of Salieri yelling "MOZART!!!" from Amadeus was the best . . . she has an incredible man-voice that she harnesses from deep within. Oh my goodness, maybe you had to be there.

I don't write much on the blog, but today is the day to do it. For those of you who know us well, I am so close to my mom that it sometimes terrifies me. Maybe it terrifies her too. I know how lucky I am to have a mom like her, and parents like mine, and our situation—my situation—has made our link stronger, and sometimes that's scary. We both know that there will be a time, hopefully, strangely, where I am well again and we live apart like typical adult mother and daughter, and we will look back on this time with nostalgia. Right now we are suspended, and we do puzzles together and watch Mad Men and she gives me leg massages, and everything, good or bad, is heightened. Everything makes me cry these days, good things more often than bad—so there's a lot of appreciating that goes on. But it's also draining, exhausting. Living in the moment is a good adage, but like anything, there can be too much of it.

My mom is doing everything for me, she has uprooted herself. My dad is living alone in MA when he is not here, and I know it's hard for him in a way I can't imagine. Andrew is back and forth as well. Here since December though, non-stop, has been my mom. She cooks, does the laundry, listens to me, sits with me in the ER, in the hospital . . . she even feeds Henry homemade food that she makes herself. Here in Pittsburgh, where she knew no one, she has made friends and found interesting things to do, always finding something to be enthusiastic about. Even writing this now is making me want to be more like her, and I feel even more thankful just putting it into words.

She has somehow found time to write every day, and has since July 1st, circling the date in red when she is done—she has remarkable follow-through with things. It has taken me over 2 months to gain 4 pounds, and I WOULD NOT have been able to do it without her. When you get evaluated for transplant, part of the evaluation is making sure you have a good support system, because it is so vital to how well you do. This might seem hard to grasp to a healthy person who thinks that ultimately, you can get through anything on your own if you really have to. I am telling you—haha—you can't. You need people, and I wouldn't be here without her.

I am also aware on a day like today how hard it must be for some people, who have to be painfully reminded each May that they don't, for whatever reason, have that relationship. It reminds me again that everybody has some kind of pain, as well as some kind of good in their life, and that none of this is a contest. As hard as it is being sick and being here, my mostly companion and I are having some laughs. There's probably a lot of people out there with great lungs, and no mummy. Everybody is just trying.

As it usually is when you love someone so much you can't put it into words, everything I have written here feels inadequate. But most of you already know what a great mummy she is, I am just here to tell you . . . that she is even better than that, and that I love her so so so much.

Happy Mother's Day!

7

THE BALCONY SUMMER

Three memories stand out from that balcony summer. We saw the blue moon, the one about which Caitlin had written five years earlier on New Year's Day: *Love you. Love when I see the new year. It's all just a weird time construct but I hope I see blue moon 2015!!*

She and I watched it from our window high on the fifteenth floor in Pittsburgh and here it is, right there on my phone: the full moon shining through a band of bright clouds, the lights of Mount Washington reflecting in the black river below. She stood tucked under my chin, and the feeling then was like the feeling now, like I am existing inside multiple dimensions as I remember how I recalled that 2010 text and our first, apprehensive trip to the city where we now found ourselves trapped inside time, waiting.

I take another look, now, at the words of that old text, black on white, and I think, *Her fingers typed out each letter.* I only copied and pasted them.

The second memory is this: Nick and Andrew in town, all

four of us sitting around after dinner, laughing over some funny thing on television. Out of our living room windows we can see fireworks over the Pirates' baseball field. Henry is tucked against my leg.

This is good, I think. *We are all together. There's not much in life that's better than this.*

In that moment I surrender to the uncertainty. I am actually euphoric with it. In that moment, I don't mind waiting one bit.

The third memory is Jess.

One weekend she flew in from San Francisco for a visit with Caitlin that fed them both. It was a joy to see them curled up on the sofa, talking and laughing and enjoying a few days' doses of normalcy.

The day Jess flew back to California, I accompanied her down to a waiting Uber. Her eyes turned bright with tears as she hugged me. It killed her to see Caitlin struggling, she said. "I just love my little buddy so much."

As I hugged her in return, I couldn't help but think about the contrast. Jess was like an ad for good health, standing so straight and strong and beautiful. How was it that some people could be so sick from birth, and others live their whole lives with no issues?

Caitlin spent most afternoons working on the Prouty Garden fight. The previous summer, waiting in Boston and confined indoors, she had felt her life to be at a standstill. Now her life had meaning, checklists. Purpose.

A GoFundMe page they created raised thousands of dollars. That summer they gathered the voices of patients, parents, and medical staff and published them.

"My son spent his final night in the garden."

"When my son was battling cancer and we were living in the hospital, that garden was the brightest spot in our darkest days."

"Often it is the last place we take our MSICU patients when we withdraw care. Parents find peace in it as it's the last place their child has been alive."

Caitlin was tenacious, but they were up against money and power. I feared magical thinking, that she was aligning her own health with the life of the garden: if the garden was saved, so, too, would she be saved.

❦

One day I experienced a bit of a scare, a squeezing in my heart that I guessed was muscular, but I didn't want to be stupid. Heart disease had killed one of my grandmothers at age fifty-two, and her son, my father, at fifty-nine.

Luckily, Andrew was arriving from the airport at any minute. As soon as he came in the door and Caitlin was in good hands, I said I was off to buy groceries.

"Please be careful driving," Caitlin said, her ritual good-bye.

At the ER, my EKG and bloodwork showed I had not had a heart attack, and everything looked okay, but I hadn't realized they would want to keep me overnight. I called Caitlin to let her know.

"I knew something was wrong! I said to Andrew, 'Something is up!'"

Now she insisted on coming to the hospital to see me and bring me dinner. I said no, I was okay, I was only grateful Andrew was there. "I really am happier knowing you're home taking care of yourself, bud."

But an hour later, in they came, Andrew pushing her wheelchair, a big brown bag on her lap containing my favorite meal from a local restaurant.

All night and into the next morning, she monitored my care via constant texts, insisting that I insist on a battery of tests now that I was there anyway, and conferring with physician friends to ensure that I got the complete cardiac workup I never would have pushed for or received on my own.

Nick was on a flight from Boston. He forwarded the email she'd sent.

How you can help: Mum needs to get that test to conclusively rule out pulmonary embolism. I need you to trust me on this and make sure you support and back me up in making sure she follows through and gets 100% clear. These residents on duty are just doing their thing which is not super vigilant. She may get tired and overwhelmed—I think she already is, and "just wants to get out of there." Trust me.

My inpatient night was horrific, with condescending residents, an attending who resented Caitlin's push for tests and snapped at me before agreeing to them, and a roommate on the other side of the curtain who spent the entire night on a commode with diarrhea.

I was Tom Hanks in *Big*, curled up and crying on a bare mattress.

It was a gift of an experience, though. The cardiac workup uncovered a hidden condition I would need to monitor for the rest of my life. More important, that miserable night gave me a personal and terrifying taste of the reality of living sick, of dependence on medical people and being at the mercy of their attitudes. Sickness in old age comes for most of us, and now I would be better prepared to deal with it.

*

Jess ran the San Francisco Nike half marathon on a bright October morning. Afterward, she texted Caitlin to say it had gone well but she'd noticed pain in her breast and could feel a lump. She said she would get it checked in Boston when she went home for Christmas.

"Jess," Caitlin said, "you have to see someone *now*."

Jess was diagnosed with stage three breast cancer on the twenty-seventh of October. Suddenly she found herself wrenched from her job and frequent visits to Kenya, and forced into the world of biopsies and PET scans and genetic testing and egg freezing.

The plan was chemotherapy for six months, followed by a lumpectomy and radiation.

I thought of how healthy Jess had looked during that visit in August. I thought of how healthy Caitlin looked whenever she took off her oxygen. They were two books you could not judge by their beautiful covers.

What were the chances that such close friends would both end up dealing with major medical issues at such a young age and at the same time?

I lay awake the night of the diagnosis, my mind ruminating on the fact of Jess and breast cancer. The world could seem random in its cruelty, but was it? Or were these life lessons these two souls had laid out ahead of time, as people like Dr. Brian Weiss would say?

Jess would write, on her own blog, "The upside is that I have been overwhelmed by the kindness of humanity."

*

11/1/2015

CAITLIN: Only a few things have ever stayed with me like *The Witches* movie did.
Another one was *The Diving Bell and the Butterfly*. I am so terrified of having a stroke like that. Locked-in syndrome. I am so so afraid of it in ways I can't even be ok with.

⁂

November, December. Dark days. Days that felt like the waiting would never end. Caitlin's Prouty Garden fight dragging into a new year and my heart pinching at the sight of her, bent over her laptop, drafting blog posts and ads and appeals.

In December, renowned biologist and conservationist E. O. Wilson appealed to the hospital: *I believe that what you plan will put you on the wrong side of history. Scientific evidence, obtained in both Europe and the U.S., support the claims made for the healing powers of natural environments adjacent to and within hospitals. The Prouty Garden has more than just great practical value in medicine. It is also a source of comfort for patients and their families. Further, it has become a symbol of those values for which Boston is famous.*

We often longed for the Prouty Garden and the balm of its existence. So many times during Caitlin's many inpatient years in Boston we'd stolen outside to the garden to plant our feet in grass or make a tiny snowman.

Exactly twice, as an inpatient at Pittsburgh, I wheeled her over to the UPMC hospital garden, an open-air platform area with some sparsely planted beds and an overpowering smell of exhaust fumes from the adjacent parking garage.

As medical help grew increasingly powerless to ease Caitlin's increasingly intolerable discomfort, Caitlin incorporated other types of healing she found to be therapeutic. More frequently, she and her cousin Sinéad, in London, communicated so that Sinéad could send what she called distance healing.

Sinéad is an intuitive, an empath, a clairsentient, a healer—there are many words for Sinéad and none fully describes her. When she was little, we laughed about her two imaginary friends, Plackie and Leenaw. She described them as two young men, one wearing a soccer jersey, the other something that sounded like the garb of a Dickensian waif. She grew up to be an empath, and years later, a fellow empath "read" her and said she saw two guides with her, one wearing a soccer shirt, the other an Artful Dodger kind of getup.

Sinéad *knows* things, and I've been witness to her initial confusion, dismissal, then growing acceptance and development of her heightened intuitive abilities. I'm not surprised when I read exposés about so-called psychics and mediums who've been caught researching and cold-reading their clients, but I also know that people like our niece do exist, people who have abilities they never asked for or even wanted.

12/22/2015

CAITLIN: Do you think it's totally paranoid to think what if the hospital or people there are so corrupt that somehow they know I've been a big part of this Prouty thing, and someone has a friend somewhere and that's why I am not getting called for transplant. Like what if they really investigate shit and they see the checks to the lawyer have come from me.

I think I've seen too many Trumbo, spotlight, suffragette movies. . . .

CAITLIN: Orange juice. Grapes. Seeds. Nuts.

Just sending reminders so I don't forget.

<hr>

9LivesNotes Post: 12/25/2015

Caitlin: "Ruby Slippers"

Caitlin here.

I wear slippers every day. After two years of waiting for transplant, my feet are softer and smoother than they've ever been. My wardrobe is an alternating cycle of loungewear. I've been wearing the same pair of worn-out, beige L.L.Bean slippers for years. A couple of months ago, I bought the red version. I'd wanted a pair for a few years now, but they sell out around Christmas. So in October—because right now I have the foresight for these kinds of things—I thought, Oh, I will buy these now, and these will be my after-transplant slippers, when I am in the hospital.

When the new ones arrived, I wanted to wear them, but I left them in the box and put them in the corner of my room.

I like astrology. It's hard to say "I believe" in astrology. I don't know what I believe in, fully, when it comes to religion or spirituality. I believe in myself, the love of my family and friends, and the idea that being kind and true feels like the most important thing in life. Astrology is fun. I have been learning about it since I was a tween—and after 20 years of it, you notice patterns that are hard to dismiss as coincidence. So I pay attention to it, I've had my chart read. I notice what happens, and what doesn't. For example, Jupiter was in Leo for a good part of my waiting time. Jupiter is the "giver of gifts and luck." I thought for sure this meant my transplant would happen. Jupiter was in Leo for a year— there was plenty of time. But Jupiter came and went. It's not like I was counting on a planet, roughly 400 million miles away, to give my tiny speck of a body a break, but how can you not think of that once you've heard it? The year did bring me a lucky break though. It wasn't until May of 2015, after being listed one year, that we found out I had been unknowingly growing something new in my lungs. Had I been transplanted before we found it and treated it, it would have put my new lungs at a much greater risk. You can't always get what you want, but . . . as the song goes.

Today December 25, all the planets in our solar system "go direct." This means they are all moving toward us, instead of away from us (when they would be retrograde). This is sort of rare— and usually happens about once a year. It's a time of opportunity; supposedly the channels are all open, ready to facilitate whatever comes down the line—everything is unstuck. Oddly this never happened in 2014—it was an off year. In fact, they haven't all been direct like they are now since January–February 2013—a full two years ago.

I've been a grinch all week, but it lifted today, as I knew it would eventually. I am always comforted by knowing the tide will change, even if the tide is just the ebb and flow of your own mood. Maybe it is the stars doing it, maybe it's the idea of the stars. Perhaps it comes from inside you the whole time. However you get there, it's like a relief and if you hang on long enough you'll *get a little glimpse of clarity and you move forward an inch, or a millimeter, or a mile.*

    Merry Christmas to everyone, whatever kind of year you are having. I hope it's good, and if it's tough, believe in yourself to get through it. And for my dear little buddy Jess, who is facing her own breast cancer diagnosis this Christmas—I hope all the people who have been so kind to me, and read this, can send some of your goodness her way. She is a light of a person, a funny little sparky bright light in my life. Here's to 2016 for both of us, for everyone!

                    ❦

For Christmas, Caitlin gave me a reading with the astrologer she'd referenced in her post, with whom she had struck up a correspondence. The astrologer didn't just read your natal chart. She provided information about your "transits," as in where you were in life right now.

My reading happened over the phone and it was cordial and insightful, a kind of lark. Afterward, the astrologer followed up with a write-up of my transits and said that if I had any questions, to just ask.

I did want clarification on a couple of points. I wrote once, then a second time to press for specifics on a particular sentence.

ME: Dealing with death? Is that what this transit means? I realize you may be speaking metaphorically, and my new novel does have a bit to do with coming to terms with the end of life, but just wondered what you meant by the choice of phrase, "dealing with death." Thank you.

ASTROLOGER: Pluto in challenging aspect to Venus can be symbolic or actual death. I do suspect there will be a death of someone close in your life (and Caitlin's) and I am also feeling that Caitlin could have a rough time of it. But that is not certain. It's all possibilities. . . . People in your life may be passing away during this time and will create an ongoing communication with you that will turn out to be a major part of your life with the SUN/Moon progressed aspect in Cancer. Perhaps your dad will be in communication with you often? Or Caitlin, if she on a Soul level lets go of her body and dies she will for sure be in touch with you and teaching you from the spiritual realms. This is not certain, of course. I do not know. However, it seems likely because the SUN/MOON progression is in the 8th house that someone important will be passing away within a year or so.

What the fuck.

8

AN UNFINISHED YEAR

It will happen when you least expect it so try not to expect it don't hear the phone ring write your book do the chores go to the gym jump on the bike pedal hard jump-rope jump-rope jump jump jump.

The rest is reward, a little bit of peace in the day. The hush of the steam room. The white mist.

The echoes.

Alone in that place I always think, *How easily I can breathe any kind of air without worry.*

Alone with the mist, I always think, *One day it must happen. One day I will forever after know the date.*

On a cold January morning the day after David Bowie died, Caitlin and I huddled on the sofa with her laptop. Together we watched *Lazarus,* Bowie's haunting last music video, released just a few days before his death.

Lazarus probably partly refers to the Old Testament story of Jesus raising Lazarus of Bethany from the dead, but the video is more complicated than a simple interpretation. It's a difficult video to watch, its opening image focused on a shadowy wardrobe, doors ajar. Fingers belonging to a dark presence creep out, then a saxophone groan drags the camera over to Bowie, writhing and partly levitating above a hospital bed. His head is wrapped in bandages, metal buttons sewn into the fabric like the shroud of a dead man crossing the River Styx. *Look up here, I'm in heaven,* he sings as the saxophone grinds down to the presence, now under his bed, its fingers crawling up the blankets toward his body.

That morning, Caitlin wrote one of her infrequent blog posts, this one about how much music meant to her. "Some precious, rare songs never, ever get old," she wrote. "They always lift you up, change your day, track the course of your life."

She went on to write about "Under Pressure" in particular, the collaboration between Bowie and Queen.

Some lyrics stand out not as the most famous lines, or even as singular, cohesive ideas, but as the part of the song that just makes your heart soar, or break. These lyrics don't behave like normal words . . . they fail to incite feeling without the song itself—that is the magic of music. It is the music, and David Bowie and Freddie, that gives you a shiver, chokes you up . . . whatever is happening, it ends up transcending words. Today, in the flood of Bowie tweets and posts, I heard the isolated lyrics for the first time and I felt that awe that I sometimes feel with really original music—a combination of, "how did someone even think to write this?" and "thank God they did."

01/10/2016

NICK: Check out the town of Ravenna in Italy and its very old church ceiling.

CAITLIN: Don't need to. It's been one of my favorite places since I was in high school. I've always wanted to go there. I love that kind of art and something about that town has always called to me.

NICK: I'm not normally into churches. I have a hard time understanding/stomaching the toll on human life to create these monuments. But at 4 this morning I was taken by its beauty and history.

CAITLIN: So what I always loved about Early Christian art was that it was so . . . early. Really the beginnings of Christianity, and thinking about what that meant is neat for me. This was years before even the crusades, the first really violent time in the name of "Christ" (well except for Christ himself obviously). So there was violence of course . . . in Rome and in the Byzantine empire. But Christianity hadn't even reached a point yet where people were "fighting in the name of the Catholic Church" etc and things were still more modest.

You can see the change in how Christ is portrayed in the art in these small churches. He's still a shepherd but he's wearing Roman robes and looks more regal. So it's the beginnings of it. . . . But it's unlikely that these religious people then were implementing awful atrocities on people.

I think the area seems beautiful and peaceful. But also something I can't really place, and don't necessarily need to figure out. I just would like to go.

There is always going to be bad in the world. I think that is what makes being good so important.

Jess mused about how fitting it would be if she and Caitlin ended up having surgery on the same day. Her lumpectomy was scheduled for April 12. And there was that "four" again; four could still mean April. A surgery more than two years after the day I'd first questioned the psychic certainly qualified as "cold."

Two years later, everything was more of an effort. Lungs, heart, blood sugar, headaches, body aches. The frigid weather didn't help. When the temperature dropped, the valves on the oxygen tanks could freeze, so she had to stay cooped up. Ten days could go by without her ever leaving the apartment. She was like Rapunzel, up there on the fifteenth floor.

On Groundhog Day, the irony was almost too stark to make jokes, but we did. *Two years! Hahaha!* Selfies with our chainsaw groundhog. I thought of my thoughts back in 2014: *Okay! Let's get this over with so our lives can get back to normal!*

Those days saw Caitlin's wait for transplant and the fight to save the garden dragging on in tandem. She used her graphic design skills to create full-page ads that would run in *The Boston Globe*.

One ad highlighted the E. O. Wilson quote about the hospital putting itself "on the wrong side of history." The ad included the names of hospital staff who had joined more than seventeen thousand protesters.

Another featured famed and beloved pediatrician T. Berry Brazelton: "Some children's ashes have been scattered in that garden. I think it should be treated as a sacred space."

A third showcased the dawn redwood tree and the words: SAVE ME.

Thomas Farragher wrote another *Boston Globe* column that began, "As I have written before, the hospital has constructed this false choice: You can either have the garden, or you can have clinical space where we will continue to save children. There is a public hearing on the proposal on Thursday at which the hospital will doubtlessly repeat a version of that argument to officials from the state Department of Public Health, whose authorization it needs to proceed."

I was nervous about the outcome. The fight was getting legal and it could not go on forever. Just like our waiting *must* end at some point.

From: Caitlin
To: Jess
Date: 2/9/2016
Subject: Late night thoughts

There have been a few times when I've been just so scared for how I am going to FEEL. It's a weird kind of anxiety because it's not being afraid of PAIN so much, or of a gross procedure, but just like "how bad can something feel and not be pain . . . ?"

The unknown misery that may come. Not imagining how you'll deal with it. I feel that way when I imagine waking up from transplant and being on a ventilator. That has been my biggest hurdle in the fear dept. Like how fucking scary will that feel. I am still working on it. . . .

But one of them, one of those feelings I've been so afraid of, is when I have gotten SVT—and I have to have this medicine to reset it called adenosine. It's not the feeling of the SVT—it's the adenosine. The first time I had it I was sort of unprepared—the situation is like an emergency and you feel bad anyway with SVT so not sure how you can be prepared. But anyway, it basically "makes you feel like you are dying"—literally—for 5 seconds. Thank God it's quick because it's really bad. It slows your heart to near stopping—hence the death feeling—so that it restarts at a normal pace hopefully. But those 5-10 seconds are indescribable. It's like your body is shutting down and you're conscious.

Anyway that was like in 2005 or something—the first time I had it—and I was so so so so so afraid to ever have it again. But eventually I had to have it again. In the past few years, many times. And at this point I have it every time I have gone to the ER for SVT—sometimes multiple times in a row.

The weirdest part is I have almost moved into a stage where I don't really mind it at all. I kind of flow with it. It still feels horrible? I guess? But I don't know anymore. It's strange because the sensation is exactly the same. I just process it differently.

There have also been times when I am just so miserable that are different from that. I remember January 2014 when I was so sick and just wanting to sit with my head in my hands. I couldn't even talk. I would procrastinate for an hour walking 3 feet to the bathroom because I didn't want to move but just lying there was painful anyway. Everything hurt. It hurt to be alive. But I couldn't sleep either. Remember when you and Alyssa came over that day to my parents, and we all sat on the couch? I wanted to die. You know what I mean—not really die—but I just felt like there was nothing not one single thing that could make me not be in misery in every way. Not lying down. Not anything to eat or drink. Not a shower. Nothing. That time is like a vacuum.

I bring both these up because the first one—the fear of how something will make you feel—is wicked scary but I realized the more I had the medicine that, like I do sometimes with needles—I could do this thing where I diffuse the feeling by getting really really close to it. I don't know if this will make sense—but it's kind of the same technique as exposure therapy that people do in cognitive behavioral stuff—i.e.—you are afraid of heights so you have to slowly go out on the balcony bit by bit to face your fear. I never liked when nurses would try to distract me from the needle. Or ask me a question while they were about to stab me. Instead I focused on it. And now it's my technique. I focus on it so intently while staying relaxed—almost like I am accepting and feeling every sensation. The pain of a needle stops being shocking "pain" and simply becomes sensation, somehow. Like everything is just sensation on a different scale. I also thought about how you'd hear that in a drunk driving accident the only person who didn't get hurt was the drunk because a drunk person doesn't brace themselves. I think when you brace yourself, you go against the grain of what is happening to you. You make it more difficult. It's more uncomfortable.

So that's one thing.

But then sometimes you're so miserable that it's all you can think about. It's a different kind of misery. Nausea. Aches. Exhaustion. It's different than pain or bizarre quick sensations. That's when crossword puzzles are good. Also download the game "two dots." I like that one for real spaced-out times. Yahtzee is ok too. But during these bad times . . . That's when your brain takes over and saves you. It goes into survival mode and doesn't let you experience really how bad it is. That's why it's so hard to imagine now. So if it is that bad—it won't be the normal you experiencing it. It will be survival Jess. And survival Caitlin is like a robotic emotionless drone haha (who makes jokes). Most of the time. Which is a good thing. So I hope you won't feel so bad that survival Jess has to kick in—but I promise she will if you do—and it's good—it's like having someone else take over for a little while. Like survival Jess was there when you got diagnosed, I am sure. . . . You've met her. You wrote about it.

Right now you're probably like half survival Jess, half regular Jess. I feel like I'm more 70/30—70 regular because things are ok right now and I'm way too used to this waiting game. Plus, nothing acute is happening to me right now.

I have no idea how you're going to feel and I am sure what I have felt is also nothing like what you might feel. I don't think you can ever really know what another person feels—even someone with the same disease. I have heard people describe CF in such different ways from me! Renu always says she felt like an elephant was sitting on her chest. I don't feel that at all. Who knows if I stub my toe and you stub your toe if we feel the same thing. I just felt like writing to you about my experiences with misery and fear—and to let you know that your mind and body are capable of incredible resilience. Something will happen, something kicks in, even if you feel so terrible that will keep you "ok" . . . even if it seems impossible now.

I love you!

⁂

At the Department of Public Health hearing, which Nick and my brother Michael attended, they read Caitlin's statement. We watched via a live feed as her written words explained who she was and what gave her the authority to speak.

> *My lung function is at 20%. I'm on oxygen 24/7. I sometimes use a wheelchair. I have a list of other complications, heart, bones, digestive problems, that stem from 32 years of chronic infection. I am in a lot of pain and discomfort. As much as I dislike listing off my ailments like this, I relay it all to illustrate that I truly am a long-time patient, and I know what it is like to be a very sick child.*

Life in the hospital is a surreal weird tunnel of heightened moments—beauty, anguish, anxiety, love, humor, dark weird humor, apathy, and clarity. That's what being stuck in a hospital, really sick, is like . . . it is the extreme emotions of life, all smashed together and turned up a notch . . . reality is distorted. You find calm in the Prouty garden, and also vitality. You remember what it is like to be part of the world, in real nature, and it's invigorating. It's special and sacred, and I feel anger towards those who claim the right to say they know what's best. I hope no one has to experience the kind of pain that some of us have, but then I also think, it is kind of a gift, to understand how sacred the Prouty is . . . and I can't make anyone "get that."

She spoke of hospital "green spaces," like the one at UPMC, and compared them to the Prouty. She pointed out that during the construction of a new building, there would be no green space at all.

A year goes by fast for a real estate developer. But there are patients who will live, and suffer, and die in that hospital during that year. What will the lack of any green space do to their health, to their spirit? What does that say about the administration's ability to make the right decisions?

Maybe it should come down to a vote. But who votes? Do the kids who have died in the garden get to vote? Do their parents? Do the doctors who have come and gone already get to vote? Does Mrs. Prouty? Do I, in Pittsburgh? There are too many people, so we have to turn to public opinion—and precedent. FOUR decades of administrations avoided razing the Prouty garden before now—a tempting half acre in crowded Longwood. Did they just forget it was there? Of course not. They knew that it was *untouchable, a thing to be preserved, an asset to their hospital. Seventeen thousand people have petitioned to save the garden. A growing force of patients, world-renowned doctors, and families have been arguing this for FOUR YEARS, saying, **guys, this is the wrong move.** The people who they are fighting against? A small group of three or four major administrators, and a board of nineteen trustees. That small group has all the power because of their position, their money, and their connections. Do those make this right?*

❧

I often hoped to hear that long-ago voice saying *Have faith* again. I did not. But close to the impossible second anniversary of her transplant listing, I was doing chest PT on her when I heard her voice, not her real voice, clearly say, *I'm dying, Mom.*

What had I heard?

In *The Mind's Eye*, the late neurologist Oliver Sacks wrote about auditory hallucinations—he'd had one himself in a moment of danger—and declared them to be an "ultimate safeguard" built into the brain.

It did not feel like a safeguard. It felt real, and it felt like a warning.

❧

In May, Katie went to a psychic. She was feeling discombobulated because she'd been pregnant with her second child but had had a late miscarriage and who knew if this stuff was true, but she was looking for any assurance, any kind at all!

The psychic picked up on her loss and said, "Oh, don't worry, that soul's coming back, it just needed to check in, the time wasn't right. You'll be pregnant soon and you'll have a girl."

Then she said, "Someone very close to you, a sister, someone close?" And she put both hands on her chest and thumped. "Something's wrong here."

"That's Caitlin," Katie said. "She's my best friend, like my sister. She's waiting for a lung transplant."

The psychic thumped her chest again and said, "It's going to be a good match." The donor would be young and healthy, she said. "An accident."

I wanted to get through this time with as much gratitude and integrity as possible, but I felt like a vulture hanging on to those words.

⁂

Caitlin's lung function declined. Her pulmonary hypertension grew worse. Her care rituals became even more complicated and time-consuming.

And the Prouty fight was faltering. The group had filed a lawsuit against the hospital, alleging that the hospital had violated state law and regulation by proceeding with construction of and fund-raising for the twelve-story facility without obtaining necessary state approval, but the hospital put up fencing in the garden and began geological boring anyway.

In June we signed on for another year on our condo.

The limbo, the uncertainty, the sameness of the days—I felt like I would combust if I had to live another year of Groundhog Day. The nagging sense of service that I'd always lived with came back, and I started volunteering again. Once a week, I read to a man with ALS.

It wasn't entirely selfless, I recognized that. Getting out of my own difficult routine and helping another person with his helped me accept what I had to cope with. And Barry became a new friend. He was a Taoist, a hawk expert, a lifelong professional photographer and all-around interesting man.

Caitlin had no such outlets, and for the first time, she sounded defeated. "It's not going to happen," she said. "We should just go home."

I said, "It will happen when we least expect it. That's what everyone says. Imagine someone in a Third World country, say, who had no chance of getting a lung transplant, and if you said to them, 'You can live in this great apartment and get a lung transplant at this great transplant center,' it would be a dream for that person. So we have to sit tight and think of that. Right?"

But it wasn't just the waiting and the garden getting her down.

Jess was facing a third surgery. After her April lumpectomy, her margins had not remained clear and she underwent a unilateral mastectomy. At a follow-up appointment, when she mentioned that some scar tissue had formed at the site of her original tumor, her surgeon examined the area and assured her that it was nothing to worry about, that there was no chance that her cancer could have returned.

But a needle biopsy proved that the cancer had returned. It was something that both of her oncologists said they had seen only once in their more than thirty years of practice. A .001 percent chance of happening. So Jess was scheduled for another mastectomy. After recovery, she would go home to Massachusetts to recuperate.

9LivesNotes Post: Father's Day 2016

Caitlin: "The Menu"

Caitlin here.

Yesterday my dad sent my mom and me a photo of a little menu he had drawn up: "How to entertain yourself when your wife is in Pittsburgh." He had gone to the Ashland farmer's market that morning—where he is a regular, making the rounds—after returning the previous night from the Vineyard, with fresh fish caught by his buddy there. The menu had smiley faces at the end of certain options. For Starters there were "Cotuit Oysters—Just Grilled :)", Mains came with a choice of greens which included the option of "Snap Peas—as is. :)" There was Rosé from Provence to drink and "Trio of homemade cheeses by French lady from farmer's market Ashland" as a finishing course. (He doesn't like sweets.)

This menu ripped my heart out of my chest. I'm an easy cry— but the "sad dad" phenomenon has always made me cry. "Sad dad" is not about dad being sad . . . it's about a dad, any dad, being sweet, vulnerable, nice, cute, making an earnest effort. I suppose anyone, anywhere making an "earnest effort" is enough to bring me to tears. Smiley faces, tryers for happiness in the face of difficulty. It all just gets me. The first time I became aware of the emotional power of "sad dad" was when I was about 10, not quite a teen but no longer a true child, and my father had secretly, without telling my mom, ordered a live Care Bear to show up at my birthday party. I was way too old for this, and when the Care Bear showed up I felt for the first time what it was to be embarrassed not only for yourself but for someone else, and wanting to protect them from feeling bad. That combination of feelings implodes inside your stomach and turns into "sad dad." I shared this feeling with my friend Katie, who of course, as with so many things, understood completely. Over the years our moms shared in our talking about the sad dad thing and we'd send pictures or share stories. It would always be sweet and small moments—a t-shirt or a gift, a big smile and a wave. They understood it with their fathers too, and other people could be sad dads, on tv or in movies, people we didn't know. Eventually, in Katie's case, she had a child and experienced sad dad double-time—sad husband, sad grandpa. Even a not-so-great-dad can elicit the feeling, so long as there is a painful moment of earnest trying, even if it fails. The complicated nature of all parental relationships—the drive we have to connect, protect, forgive, we are all vulnerable to that. The resulting feeling on our parts ends up being one of wanting to hug them and cry . . . and of course they are always baffled. It seems like pity, I am sure. No one wants to be labeled "sad" something. I have seen Katie, or my mom or dad or Andrew look at my small frame (which doesn't seem small to me), squeeze me and say, "Oh Kitten" and I think, "What? Don't oh Kitten me, I'm doing just fine." . . . No one wants to be the painful one, tugging at people's heartstrings. But we are, and thank goodness for that, because just as everyone wants to feel loved and protected, I think they also want to do the same for someone else.

My dad has spent his life providing for me, and subsequently protecting me. At 32, I am not married yet or having kids, but waiting for a lung transplant and still dependent on my parents. I am like the family doctor around here, watching their diets and advising them on prescriptions, checking moles, doing all the worrying. Maybe it is the one way I can protect them all, until I can stand on my own and become independent. Maybe that's where sad dad really comes from: a need to protect. I love him so much, and I suppose the things we love we want to protect, even in situ-

ations when we are not in the role of protector. My dad and I have a great time together; there are certain specific emotional moments where, despite my closeness with my mom, I find myself reaching out desperately to my dad. I am not even sure if he knows it. Perhaps they are why we chose each other in this life. We clash too, and it has made us have to try harder to achieve the friendship we now enjoy. We are a lot alike, and I think two people who are so alike do best if one is not so dependent on the other.

My dad is complicated—unafraid to change. My mom once pointed out that if he sees something he doesn't like in himself, he will and can change it . . . which is pretty rare. It is true. I like to think I have inherited that characteristic. My dad always makes everything look beautiful—even if it's just a snack of cheese and crackers, or rocks arranged on a beach, or items on a table while we're waiting for dinner. I did not inherit that as much. He is an artist at heart who sees a unique way of combining things in everything he looks at. Lately he has been sending me cards with birds on them. My grandfather, his dad, whom they called "Gigli" (after the famous Italian tenor) because of his lovely singing voice, was a milkman who kept birds. I love birds too, like my grandfather. My dad and I seek common ground. We keep up our earnest effort, because we love each other, and of course, now, I have tears in my eyes.

I dropped an oxygen tank on my foot and broke a toe. For the next couple of weeks, every morning, Caitlin carefully cleaned the purple gash and applied a fresh bandage, taking great pleasure in being able to be the one on the giving end of care.

One morning I was fretting about my new novel and my sense that I hadn't done enough with my life, that time had passed, does pass, and will always pass too quickly. I felt behind in my career.

"Oh, Mom." She waved at me with an exasperated gesture that said, *Don't you get it?* "You think all this is important, but all that really matters is loving people and being kind."

⁂

From: Caitlin O'Hara
To: Jess
Date: June 29, 2016
Subject: Survival

I figure you more than anyone appreciate honesty and genuine straight talk. So—

1.   My survival rate, 5 years after transplant is technically 50%. That's without b. cepacia—the bacteria that is the reason I am here at UPMC. There aren't really any stats for it that matter because there are so few people so there are no real studies. Some people do well. Some people just don't at all. Most all people survive the operating table and one year. But five-year survival drastically drops. After transplant, CF people often seem so happy because life before not being able to breathe sucked so much—and it gives the false impression that everything is just "fixed." But many people who don't have CF who get transplanted for other reasons say life is just as hard after. Complications galore. As they say, you trade one disease for another. I am not saying this because it's a comparison.... A "look how bad I have it too." I am saying it because I want you to KNOW that there was a time when this knowledge was impossible for me to swallow.

It seemed like hell, I thought living through it would be hell. But although I've had moments of hell (haven't we all?) I can honestly say that my life is NOT hell, and I say that with the complete acceptance that I could never end up getting married or doing much. That sounds so depressing to people so that's why I don't talk about it. But it's not like I'm just "at peace" with my illness. I'm just saying I still exist. I get excited for things. I have hope and I look forward to stuff. Because soon your brain and body adjust. We all have no idea when we are going to die. Some girl on St. John died yesterday on a moped. Some pretty 26-year-old girl and it was her birthday. The day before we probably would've been jealous of her photos and now she's dead and we're alive. THE MIRACLE OF HUMAN BEINGS IS THAT WE ARE ALL ABLE TO GO ON LIVING DESPITE THE CERTAINTY THAT WE WILL DIE. I kind of love that. So, just like you felt happy before—you will feel happy again. Because you don't know what will happen. You just never had to confront it before—but you didn't know before either! Logic doesn't always work to make you feel better right away—but stick it in your brain and it will work behind the scenes. . . .

2.   I see people go through transplant in ways that I would never go through. They're sad all the time. But then I realize they're sad after transplant too. And before! Every bit of advice you get from someone is filtered through their own life. It's so important to remember that and not let the things people say stick in your craw as fact. Imagine if all the fears YOU have right now stuck in someone else's mind as fact! You would be like . . . "Oh no I didn't mean it! I was just a mess at that time." Anyway—don't listen to anyone who tells you "You just have to accept that life is shitty." LIFE ISN'T SHITTY. It's better than the alternative. You're not dead. We're not dead. People go through way worse and create joy. Seek those stories out, Jess. The guy with ALS who writes a book even though he's paralyzed. The people who lose their

entire families in concentration camps and go on to say, "Life is incredible, I am happy." All of that is possible. I promise you. I feel it every day. And I know it's easy to find loopholes—like maybe it's easier for me because I have Andrew. And yes it would suck if we broke up but I don't doubt that I'd be back to this happy place again soon.

***

"Whenever I look at pictures from the last ten years," Caitlin said, "I can remember exactly how I felt." She was scrolling through her computer's photo library and when I glanced at the screen, she looked great in every picture.

She pointed at one where she was hilariously laughing, wearing a striped blue dress, out somewhere in the city. "I remember that night. I was desperately hoping that everyone would want to take a taxi."

Another one, from Cape Cod: "I wanted to run down that cliff like everyone else and jump and dance around the sand and party on the beach but all I could think was, how will I climb back up?"

9

HOMESTRETCH

Heather and Caitlin were the same age and they both had CF. They became social media friends via a private Facebook group for people associated with the UPMC lung transplant program. The other members were mostly older people, in need of transplants because of COPD and other more recent ailments. Although Heather lived less than an hour away, they couldn't meet in person—the chance of exchanging bacteria was too great. The six-foot caution that the pandemic forced onto the world has long been a rule for CF people: to avoid cross-infection they must stay a minimum of six feet away from each other. But they texted constantly and I got a strong sense of Heather's sweet soul. One day a package arrived in the mail—homemade cookies she had sent to cheer Caitlin.

When Caitlin first mentioned her new friend, she remarked that Heather had already been waiting three years, and was also tiny, with O+ blood. But her score was much lower than Caitlin's, by a good ten points. "She's not as sick as me," Caitlin said. "She's able to carry her oxygen on her back."

But in July, Heather got sick enough to be admitted, then readmitted. As she worsened, her score jumped, becoming higher than Caitlin's. Caitlin knew that while Heather and who knew how many other small, O+ people were waiting, she would not be called. "It's not going to happen," she said. "Let's just go home. We can set up the medical jet service if I get called. I can't spend another summer in this city, waiting."

So I packed up the car and Henry and drove us the 551 miles back to our home in Massachusetts.

The first week home she felt well enough to spend some much-needed alone time with Andrew, some immersion in the world of the living. She got her wish to walk on a beach again and texted a photo of the two of them, oxygen tanks slung over Andrew's shoulder. Big smiles. *You can't tell*, she wrote, *but I'm crying with happiness.*

She was also able to see Ahmet Uluer. He told her he'd never expected she would have to wait so long and that he felt terrible about it. He said that there was a new transplant team at the Brigham and he wanted to petition them to list her.

This was cautiously good news. Late in the game but worth a try, of course. She asked him to hold off until she drafted a letter of her own to accompany his petition.

A few weeks into that trip home, she grew weaker, more breathless, and began coughing up a lot of blood. She returned to spending much of the day in bed, and as I went up and down the stairs with trays and meds, I despaired at the fact that a full year and a half later, she was still sick in that bed, still in desperate need of a transplant.

One morning I brought up her inhaled meds and breakfast. "Oh, man," she said, "I had horrible nightmares last night!"

"So did I," I said. "I dreamed we were packing the car for Pittsburgh."

"Ha," she said. "You don't know nightmares until you're dreaming you're traveling down the River Styx."

⁂

While I was packing up for the drive back to Pittsburgh, I came across something I'd saved ten years earlier. I had once lurked on an astrologers' forum, where one of the practitioners struck me as bright and very good. I had emailed her a quick question about Caitlin. She ended up responding at length, gratis.

First, I need to tell you that the prime focus of Caitlin's chart is her sixth house. For all intents and purposes, she has 4 out of 5 of what I call the "god" planets there. The god planets are the planets that represent energy we think of as coming from God, as opposed to those energies we ordinarily think of as "human." And 3 out of those 4 were, until recently called "malefic" . . . Pluto, Saturn, Uranus. That is way too much energy for one house, especially one having to do with health.

She then told me that Caitlin was lucky to have survived the year she was eleven, that there had been great stress on her from several angles in her chart.

In another journal, I located my account of that "soul reading" Caitlin had had done around the same time.

July 10, 2009 *At the end of Caitlin's reading, during which she had revealed nothing about herself or her beliefs, she told the reader about the recurring "Nazi" nightmares she has had for much of her life.*

The reader assured her that these dreams did not mean she had been a Nazi. "You could not be bad! You had a life in that time, but it wasn't Germany. It was Czechoslovakia. You were a musical prodigy, literary, from a cultured family. You were killed at age eleven." Then she asked, "Did something happen to you in this life at eleven?"

(The whole time Caitlin was telling me this, my entire body was full of prickles and I began to cry.)

Caitlin said yes, she was eleven when she became so ill and had her lobectomy and all the resulting complications. The woman said that often a soul will reenact an earlier trauma at the anniversary age.

The musical prodigy part was also interesting because when Caitlin was young, she took flute lessons. She played so well and read music so effortlessly that her music teacher thought she practiced all the time. She never practiced. In fact, her whole soul reading had been about musical lives and how now, for many reasons, her soul type now associated music with trauma.

July 11, 2009 *So, just to do it, I Googled "pianist, child prodigy, Czechoslovakia, killed."*

And the first hit was about a book about 1940s musicians, Music in Terezin, 1941–1945. *Google had highlighted this passage: "Her family moved back to Czechoslovakia where the five-year-old Edith started her musical studies. As a child prodigy of eleven . . ."*

A few years earlier, I had published a short story in the *North American Review*. It was about a prodigious musician named Edith.

Now, rereading that 2009 journal in 2016, I recognized *Music in Terezin* as a book I had recently purchased in Pittsburgh and had been using to research my new novel. I did not remember that I had previously heard of it.

I was impressed by these synchronicities. They seemed meaningful and comforted me, as if they were some kind of assurance that yes, we were on the right path.

I sent Caitlin the passages from 2009. She responded,

I remember she asked if music was important to me. It was hard to answer. From an outsider's view—I am not a musical person. That makes me sad. Inwardly . . . I don't know how to say that music is everything to me . . . it is my life's blood, the only thing that can uplift my soul. I don't even play an instrument though.

Back in Pittsburgh, I walked into Caitlin's room the morning of September 3. She was reading something on her phone, her eyes full of tears. "Heather is on ECMO," she said.

ECMO is short for Extracorporeal Membrane Oxygenation. When a patient is connected to ECMO, her blood flows through tubing to an outside mechanism that oxygenates the blood and removes carbon dioxide before pumping it back into the body. ECMO is life support. The system requires constant, careful monitoring, carries many risks, and can't be relied on for more than a few days, a week or so at the most.

I said a prayer for Heather's kind soul, assuming the worst. I didn't see how anyone could survive ECMO plus a transplant.

I'm not sure why I had the distinct thought *Thank God this isn't going to happen to us.* Because Caitlin was increasingly rating her days as twos or threes. When it got to the point that she needed me to blow-dry her hair, because holding up the hair dryer exhausted her, she was admitted to the hospital for a two-week cleanout.

❦

In September, Katie and her husband opened the gender-reveal envelope from their ob-gyn.

They were having a girl, as the psychic Katie visited had said, and as anyone could have guessed with a fifty-fifty chance of being correct. But still.

I wanted reassurance, any kind at all. I decided to contact Alicia, the psychic from the 2014 social club party, to schedule a phone reading. On the phone with her, I provided some background about that previous, ten-minute reading and how I'd asked about the timing of the transplant and she'd said it had been "cold."

She said, "So it just never happened?"

I explained that a person had to wait for the right donor and one had no way of knowing when that would happen and that we were still waiting.

"Ohhhh, I see," she said.

She explained that she was shuffling her cards to receive beneficial energy and all that and asked a few more questions and then said, "So this is talking about the transplant stuff. Serious business here. So I'm going to start fresh. What do we need to hear about Maryanne's daughter Caitlin's transplant, any timing information, information in general about when, what, how all of this is going to transpire."

"So how long has she been waiting? A few years?"

"Two and a half."

"So right now, the first cards I get are not even slowed down, they're stopped, it's very quiet, new moon, very dark, we don't know what's happening, and then I get a rush, like suddenly something's going to happen out of nowhere. This information I'm receiving may not be completely accurate but typically it is. The cards' story that's coming out is a very dark period, hopeful/hopeless waves, back and forth, a down period, with expectations but nothing happening, it feels like it comes through very quickly and suddenly, without any warning, almost like it's unfair."

Her voice sharpened. "Has it already happened? Like it's come through and then not happened?"

"No, but that can happen. It does happen."

"I feel like there's a disappointment, looks like it's all happening then turns out there's a wrong match or something, and it doesn't happen. I know you said that hasn't happened already but it almost feels like that's in the past. Okay. So these are all really positive cards, saying it IS going to happen, I feel like it's going to happen in a twelve-month period. I see the Magician here, I see the Queen, it feels like a full circle. I'm counting the full circle from March, I'm feeling like it's going to be around the winter period.

"Somehow you make it happen, or she makes it happen, it's not really your will but it feels like it is, because there's so much *push*, and it's oh . . ." She exhaled. "It's pretty scary."

She didn't speak for a moment. "These transplants are pretty scary, but these are usually successful, right?"

"They can be. They often are."

I sat with my heart beating like mad, and even now, reading the transcription, I can't relisten to the actual recording because I don't want to hear what I didn't want to hear that day. A shift in her voice. Reluctance to continue.

"It just feels really scary, that's nothing new, I'm sure."

From: Caitlin O'Hara
To: Mom
Date: 9/10/2016
Subject: Songs

Mummy. If I'm ever sedated or in any kind of subconscious unconscious state—but stable or whatever—please make sure you play music. Over and over again I'm reminded how it "brings me back to life" . . . so it seems crazy that if I were to be out of it or really sick and have no control, that there would be no music. It could really help get me better! But I don't want to be at the mercy of what someone else plays. You probably know better than anyone at least. But I have compiled two lists. This lists music that is also good to play when I'm getting better from transplant. Or if I'm really sick. I realized it's easier if I tell you now and you can make a playlist and have it. But it's only for dire times. I listen to this music otherwise and I don't want you to just break out the playlist on like, a week like this or something. Maybe you will never have to use it except like right after TX :) But . . . if it were a time when I couldn't put music on myself. That is a good benchmark for when to use.

The first list is inspirational music. Like if I am in a coma or need to get out of whatever I am in. Or if I'm just despondent and lost hope. If things are really hard. I'm really miserable. The atmosphere for these has to be right though and obviously some songs are more raucous so—u would have to gauge. Like a time of focus and when u can listen to the music. We can talk about this if you want. It feels weird to type it.

List 1:
Roll me away bob seger
We didn't start the fire

Thunder road (both versions—slow one too)
Born to run
Gypsy—fleetwood mac
The boxer
And she was
Dancing in the dark
Do you believe in magic? (Random. The lovin spoonful)
Let it be
Losing my religion
Southern cross
One U2
If I ever lose my faith
Under pressure

List two are songs I find comforting and relaxing and can be played whenever. Comforting. But don't overdo any of it please! Obviously this is all hypothetical :)

List 2:
Copperline
Danny's song
Eyes of the world
Let it be
Losing my religion
Right down the line
Just like this train
Ramble on rose
Rocky raccoon
Southern cross
Still haven't found what I'm looking for
Where the streets have no name

Not a list, but: The refuge of the roads—Joni

*this is a special song. You can only play very sparingly or it will lose its powers. Like once or twice a year.

It was interesting to go through my music and make this list and identify the songs among MANY favorite songs that get to a certain spot in my soul.

On the morning of September 27, I was at my desk in my room when I heard Caitlin shout, "Heather got lungs!"

I ran down the hall. Caitlin was sitting up in bed reading her phone, relief and joy all over her face.

Heather had survived ECMO.

Heather got lungs!

She had waited forty-two months.

The one thing I can't do is think too much about the Prouty Garden. I fill up with too much blind fury.

While Caitlin was in the hospital, despite concerns raised by the Massachusetts Health Policy Commission, and the objections raised by thousands, the Department of Public Health recommended approval of the $1 billion expansion of Children's Hospital without much analysis of the consequences. The group vowed to continue fighting, but there had been a shift.

When Caitlin was released from the hospital, she sought to get her mind off the negative. She began to draft the letter for Dr. Uluer to incorporate into his planned petition to list her for transplant in Boston at the Brigham.

She rented a motorized scooter, desperate for a bit of independence.

And she asked me to drive her over to the artsy side of the city. She wanted to buy a guitar. At the shop, I sat to one side, admiring, as always, her lack of self-consciousness as she adjusted her oxygen and asked questions and tried out different models, ultimately deciding on a small Recording King.

At home, she enrolled in an online class and began practicing every day in the late afternoon.

"Is this bothering you?" she always asked.

"I enjoy it," I always said. And I did. I found the repeated chords soothing as I folded laundry or chopped ingredients for dinner. I can still feel that sense of contentment, the tranquility.

The memory is almost too much to bear.

⁕

I was checking into the fitness center at the nearby hotel when a staff member approached me, waving a piece of paper. A mother and daughter in our exact circumstances were staying in the hotel, she said. They were from LA. The daughter needed a lung transplant, and only Pittsburgh had agreed to evaluate her. The mother would love to talk to me.

I was inside the locker room changing into my workout gear when a young woman emerged from the shower stalls wearing a robe and towel turban and wheeling an oxygen tank. In addition to the oxygen tubing on her face, IV tubing ran from a port in her chest to an oh-so-familiar portable medicine infusion ball.

Cystic fibrosis affects digestion, and most people with the disease have had their growth stunted, but occasionally you meet a tall person with CF, and Mallory was one of them. I guessed her to be nearly six feet tall. My first thought was, *She won't have to wait too long.*

Mallory was lovely, with warm, intelligent eyes and an easy, engaging manner. We exclaimed over the coincidence of meeting. She, too, cultured the virulent cepacia that Caitlin cultured. The superbug can sometimes cause constant fevers in certain people, and that, unfortunately, was happening to Mallory. She had been on IV antibiotics to keep the fevers at bay, nearly nonstop, for the past year.

After my workout, Caitlin was to meet me at the spa entrance. This was an independent first, thanks to the freedom her new scooter now offered. I met up with her just as Mallory's mother appeared in the waiting area. A staff member introduced us, and Caitlin was able to say hello and offer to text Mallory.

The mother and I met in the hotel lobby the next morning. She was in the overwhelmed phase. Mallory would imminently need a transplant. Pittsburgh was their only hope. If accepted at UPMC, making the move from LA would be even harder than our move had been. At least Boston was a day's drive away, and BOS–PIT flights were nonstop and brief.

She asked me a barrage of quick-fire questions, then blurted, "They might die!"

I flinched. "Don't say that! This works. Transplant works. I know so many good stories."

But she had stories, too. And not all of them were good.

I almost said, *Don't go.* But it was one of those bad feelings you can't really justify and they would have gone anyway. Andrew and Caitlin had tickets to see a comedy show at the University of Pittsburgh.

They were running late and it was rainy and windy and when Caitlin got out of the car, the wind caught her breath and she started "stacking breaths"—meaning she couldn't get air and her O$_2$ saturation started going down ... down ... down. It was all happening so quickly that it was hard for Andrew to understand that something serious and terrifying was happening. She knew she would pass out and managed to say "emergency." Fortuitously, the show was close to the hospital, and Andrew was able to run down Cardiac Hill to the ER and return with help.

The stress on her body had caused her white blood cell count to jump, and her oxygen saturation had likely been in the 60 percent range. You never want to be below 88; healthy people are 95 to 100 percent. She remained in a compromised state after the episode, and was admitted for another two-week cleanout.

October transitioned to November and there was the death of Leonard Cohen, a divisive presidential election, earlier sunsets, darker days.

"Why haven't you been practicing your guitar, bud?" I asked.

"It's getting too hard to sit up and hold it," she said.

I never wanted her to see my heart when it broke, so I cast around for something positive to say. But she had begun to need help with everything. Reaching for a sweater in her closet. Tying a slipper lace that had come undone. Unscrewing a bottle cap.

One day, she began to cry. "I'm sorry," she said. "I'll take care of you someday, Mummy."

More turning away of the head. More breaking of the heart as I steadied my voice and said, "Oh, buddy, don't worry about it. I'm just so happy I can help you."

She had her monthly clinic appointment on November 2, and the good thing about her decline and higher oxygen needs meant that her score would have to go up.

Except it didn't. Every few days during the next two weeks, as her oxygen consumption soared, I would ask, "Did you hear from your coordinator yet?"

Coordinators cannot legally change a person's score, rightly so, without documented, supporting materials, and Caitlin's coordinator was waiting for some test or other, Caitlin said. But she was getting frustrated.

Meanwhile, Dr. Pilewski had given her something called an emergency non-rebreathing mask that she could use, when necessary, with a second tank to deliver supplemental, higher concentrations of oxygen.

On a scale of 1 to 10, most days of the week were now 1s. She began desatting as soon as she moved, had to crank the regular concentrator up to its limit and use the emergency non-rebreather more and more often. She was constantly asking me for Reiki and for leg massages. From London, Sinéad tuned in and focused on specific ailments with uncanny accuracy. But there was only so much comfort that massages and energy work could provide. She needed lungs.

I kept asking, "Has your score changed yet?"

"I wrote to her again," she said. "I don't know what's going on."

She was in charge of herself, had been for years, but I was getting irritated. I offered to call, get the ball rolling.

She said no. She was sure the score would change any day.

Should I have insisted? Would it have changed anything? Probably not, but it was ludicrous that her score remained unchanged when she could barely function.

I was washing her hair all the time now and trying to blow it dry but it was a constant tangle, stripped of moisture from all the medicines she took. You got one portion untangled, then moved to another part, and the part you had just untangled snarled up again.

She had always taken pride in her long hair but now she wanted to cut it.

Some of her close friends in Boston got in touch with me. They wanted to pay to send her Boston hair stylist down to cut and color her hair.

We organized it for Sunday afternoon, November 13. Caitlin was grateful and excited at the thought of having her hair look nice, but nervous, too. She was afraid she would feel so sick that she would be unable to sit through it.

I reassured her I would make everything work, and on Sunday, the stylist flew in with a suitcase full of supplies and got to work.

I kept a hawk eye on her the whole time, anticipating her needs, because I knew she wouldn't speak up if she was having difficulty or required help.

That night, she was so happy, so grateful. "I was so nervous that I wasn't going to be able to get through it," she said. "You watched me the whole time and made it work. Thank you so much."

It was evening, two days later. She was supposed to show up for a six fifteen cardiac catheter appointment the next morning, to determine whether her pulmonary hypertension had worsened enough that it might help increase her lung allocation score.

For Caitlin to get out of the house comfortably, she needed a good night's sleep and a couple of hours to eat, do her nebulizer treatments, take her meds, and brace herself for physical activity.

Now, with her deteriorating before my eyes, a 6:00 a.m. appointment for something as invasive as a cardiac catheter procedure was clearly ridiculous.

I went into her bathroom, where she was sitting in the tub waiting for me to wash her hair. Her iPhone sat on the floor, playing music.

She didn't acknowledge my presence. Her eyes were flat and hopeless in a way I'd never seen.

I realized what was playing. Joni Mitchell, "The Refuge of the Roads."

"Hey bud," I said, my casual tone concealing my terror, "come on. Joni wouldn't want you to be listening to this." I picked up the plastic cup to rinse her hair.

"I can't." She shut her eyes as if she might pass out. "I need to lie down."

I helped her into bed and went straight to my desk to email Dr. Pilewski. "I am beside myself . . ." I began.

10

OUR HUMAN ASSUMPTIONS

11/17/2016

CAITLIN: My score is 70.

MARYANNE: Oh wow

What happened

CAITLIN: Dr. Hayanga came in.

Because of my oxygen.

MARYANNE: Oh my god. Thank god.

CAITLIN: Idk if I'm going to do the cath. It may be moot point now.

MARYANNE: Right. What did Hayanga say

CAITLIN: He was optimistic. Very. He was like we expect to get offers.

It made me nervous!! Nervous to be hopeful.

Andrew says we HAVE to be hopeful

MARYANNE: We ARE hopeful.

It WILL happen.

9LivesNotes Post: November 20, 2016

Caitlin: "Any Colour You Like"

You can't always get what you want. Blah blah blah. Deep thoughts and Pink Floyd. There is no dark side of the moon really matter of fact it's all dark.

I'm not the first person to be sick and I won't be the last, but here we are.

Update needed.

Free association is about the only thing I have a mind to do right now and so I'll try to pull it together into something comprehensible.

If you've ever been in a major hospital recently there's this channel called C.A.R.E. that just shows pictures of nature while music plays. Apparently there's scientific evidence that just looking at a picture of a "vista" can relax you. Sometimes I lie there and watch that channel and think about the word "teeming" because that's all that keeps popping into my head. This planet is surrounded by rocky and fiery and gas-laden planets and yet ours is teeming TEEMING—with colors and creatures and millions of upright humans communicating. If you think about that for long enough and stare long enough into the bubbling rapid or the alpine peak on the screen you can get to that state of wonder for a second . . . and be like . . . pretty ok with everything.

Are you in control?

This is a question my dad often poses to me, and Andrew, during trying hospital times. Perhaps my mother gets it too, though I suspect not. It's his way, I think, of assuring himself and us that we are in control of things when he's not around. He likes to be in control. I like to be in control. I am in control as much as anyone can possibly be in my situation. Sometimes too much. I can't control the big event, the most important thing; no one can. Control is the word of the day, the year—for me—and the country it seems too. Control is elusive. Dangerous. People freak out when they lose it.

Tolstoy had an existential crisis where he couldn't figure out how to have faith . . . and decided the only logical thing he could do was to kill himself—He spiraled out of control . . . he couldn't think himself out of the problem of living, the meaninglessness of life, and the uncertainty of faith. He thought that if life had no meaning, which his reasonable mind believed because he could not prove the opposite, then the brave thing to do would be to end it. But he did not want to kill himself at all. He finally found his kernel of faith exactly right in front of him. His desire not to die, to keep on living despite the fact that he KNEW he was going to die, was a kind of miraculous leap of faith that we all do every day when we wake up. He figured the fact that faith even exists at all makes it a truth in and of itself. And he went on. (You can read this in his "A Confession").

So the basic details of my situation are things I know people want to know . . . I'm so grateful I have so many people that care for me and my family, so here they are. I went into the hospital last Wednesday because I'd reached a new low of shortness of breath, due in part obviously to my lungs but also to my pulmonary hypertension which is more severe now. My increased oxygen needs have now boosted my score way up to 70. It was 47/48 for the past 2.5 years. I cried with relief that there had finally been a shift. Just days and weeks before had been, as yet, my lowest point. For the sake of transparency and for anyone reading this who might be sick too and think a lot of people make it look easy—trust me—we all fake it. Here's what low looks like—I was sitting in the bathtub while my mom washed my hair. On

10 liters of oxygen with a rescue tank next to me to supplement. The day before I went into the hospital I couldn't even do that. Physical anxiety attacks every day. Extreme body aches. It's hard to pray for yourself. Or ask for things for yourself. But that day I screamed in my mind to whoever was listening to please help me out because I couldn't find my little ball of fiery strength any-more . . . and I can always find it.

Yet just last Sunday—I took this picture. Three of my most dearest buddies—Jacqui, Kenley, and Allison—arranged for my awesome Boston hair stylist, Alex, to fly down and completely change my hair. It had become a huge tangled yellow mess that I didn't have the energy to even comb, never mind color or cut. She came to the apartment and I cut 10 inches off and went closer to my natural color. It was so perfect and such perfect timing— because now I can have dirty hospital hair and it looks like a chic conscious fashion choice with my ripped tees. My point is—I don't look like someone sobbing in the bathtub gasping for air in this picture—but I am. Everyone struggles beyond their photos. But the world is meant to be hard and difficult and beautiful. Maybe it's easy to say this from where I sit—I am one lucky duck—I have a great family and great care, a stylist who fuck-ing flies in. I still suffer and it still sucks. But there is so much suffering in the world . . . so much. My belief though at least is—the world was not meant to always be fair or fun or easy. The world is teeming with life, and death, and pain, and Don-ald Trump even haha. We just have to keep living. Step back. We are just tiny beings. There are lobsters living at the bottom of the ocean for over a hundred years. They have just been sitting down there through all of our lives and wars and lives before us. We aren't that much different from lobsters really if you pull back a little. All part of this teeming painful wonderful world where so much is just luck. But we can choose to be kind, and to keep trying—we have the power.

"There is a crack in everything. That's how the light gets in."

—LEONARD COHEN

Two days before Thanksgiving, late in the day, about 6:00 p.m.

The three of us—me, Andrew, and Nick—were lounging around Caitlin's room, idly focused on our phones. Caitlin's nurse knocked, a funny little smile on her face. "Caitlin, your coordinator's been trying to call you."

We all looked at each other. Caitlin picked up her phone and I thought,

This is how it happens. This is how it finally happens.

It was an offer, but our relief was soon tempered. It was not an optimal offer. It was an "*ex vivo* perfusion" situation, whereby lungs that would not otherwise be suitable for transplant are treated with the hope of rejuvenating them and making them viable for a recipient. Because donor organs are so scarce, ex vivo perfusion broadens the pool of potential donor organs.

The surgeons have a moral obligation to never make offers they do not consider good, so Caitlin accepted the offer, as her transplant team advised.

The perfusion process was going to extend what always was already a long wait time to find out if surgery would be a "go." We wouldn't know anything until the next day, late morning at the very earliest. Dr. D'Cunha, the head surgeon who would perform the surgery, advised us all to get a good night's sleep.

Andrew stayed in the hospital with Caitlin. Nick and I went back to our apartment, where I stood in the living room overlooking the city lights. I had looked at these lights for nearly a year and a half of nights, wondering *when?* And now, tomorrow at this time, Caitlin might have new lungs.

⁂

Dr. D'Cunha wanted her in the CTICU so that she could be quickly transferred to the OR if surgery went forward. We were told to gather up all of her things, since she would not be returning to the room postsurgery.

It's at this point in the remembering that I let myself imagine a different outcome. Nick and Andrew pack her belongings into our car and I head down to sit by her bed in the ICU bay. We talk, we wonder, we wait. It's all we can do. The guys show up not long afterward and we are back to the hanging around that we are so accustomed to, all of us masked and gloved and gowned, using phones and books and idle conversation to help pass the time, but the atmosphere is expectant, charged. Everything for the last three years has pointed us toward this situation. Any moment, we hope to see Dr. D'Cunha walk in with "it's a go" news.

On the dry-erase board, under TODAY: the shift nurse has written:

New lungs! ☺

Caitlin is nervous, but outwardly calm. Hopeful. Cracking little jokes. Sitting up in the bed, holding Andrew's gloved hand. I have a photo of the two of them. They are in profile, her looking up at him, him looking down at her, and there is so much in that photograph. Apprehension. Courage. Love.

The clock on the wall ticks 9:00 a.m., 10:00 a.m., 11:00 a.m., and Dr. D'Cunha arrives with news that surgery is a go and she's whisked off to the OR and we move to one of the family rooms to wait for updates and hours pass and then she's out and the surgery was a bit rough but it all went well and she's recovering as expected and already my mind is moving forward—a few days in the ICU then the move to the step-down unit, then back to the medical floor and the baby-step, day-by-day recovery, a discharge by Christmas, Christmas with new lungs.

But of course that is not what happens. In fact, she waited so long that morning, with no food or drink, that it took a great physical toll. Late in the afternoon, Dr. D'Cunha emerged through the ICU doors, the regret on his face such bitter disappointment. Only one lung was viable, and Caitlin, like all patients with two infected lungs, needed two, and soon after, I wrote a brief paragraph of a post to inform everyone that Caitlin had experienced her first "dry run."

Back on the medical floor, she was assigned a new room at the far end of the hall, quieter and more private but far from the nurses' station, which always made me nervous. Out-of-sight patients are sometimes forgotten.

Nick and I went to work making the new room homelike and cozy with Christmas lights tacked around the dry-erase board, a small, twinkling tree in the window, and pictures of family, friends, and Henry on the walls.

I went home and changed into the clothes I would normally wear for a holiday. A dress and uncomfortable shoes instead of my jeans and Merrells. I packed up the dinner I'd prepared earlier and decorated an oversize lacquered tray with festive linens and a cute little ceramic turkey.

After dinner, as usual these days, she asked me for Reiki. Now, though, she told me exactly where she needed it. *My head*, she said. *My feet. Behind my right shoulder.*

Then she said, "Listen, all of you," addressing the three of us. "I need ferocious positivity from everyone." And I said, "Yes. Let's think ahead. Let's make a list."

It was time to buy new pillows. Toiletries. Nothing posttransplant could be contaminated by the cepacia from pretransplant, lest it infect the new lungs.

And how about new slippers for fun? They were back-ordered on L.L.Bean, but we ordered red scuffs, where when you put your feet together, the design on each foot formed the black silhouette of a cat.

I was in Caitlin's room when Mallory's mother texted me from California. She said that Mallory's transplant coordinator, a man named Larry, had put them in touch with the family of a young woman with CF who'd just had a transplant at UPMC. They were also from Massachusetts and they were in the hospital right now and did I want to talk to the mother?

I met the mother in the cafeteria on the top floor. It turned out we had met years ago at Boston Children's and she remembered us, remembered Caitlin's lobectomy. Their house in Massachusetts was only two towns over from ours. I was surprised and disappointed that Caitlin's coordinator had not already suggested this introduction. In fact, her coordinator had not reached out to Nick or me since Caitlin had been hospitalized with her high score.

Amanda did not culture cepacia. Her CF center was in New Haven, and she could have been transplanted pretty much anywhere. But her mother had done her research and concluded that too many transplant centers cherry-picked their patients, taking the ones most likely to have easier surgeries and recoveries and make it past the magic "one year" survival mark, and thus keep their success rate statistics high.

She said that they had moved here in the summer, when Amanda's score was 70. She'd immediately had two dry runs and they'd thought transplant was imminent. Then—nothing. August, September, October as she worsened and her LAS score climbed. Amanda was near death, her score in the 90s when she was transplanted the first week of November.

During those critical weeks, Amanda's mother even went so far as to purchase billboards in states where there were fewer patients waiting, in the hopes that a donor family might know that somewhere, a petite young woman named Amanda was in desperate need of O+ lungs.

A direct donation can bypass the strict UNOS rules and go straight to the recipient.

But billboards? "Wow," I said. "That seems so desperate."

"You don't know desperation until you're in the CTICU on ECMO with days to live."

I was listening on the outside, but inside I was shrinking. I didn't want to hear this. I was grateful Caitlin was stable and that the surgeons were actively fielding offers.

❦

Is Caitlin feeling better? Is Caitlin still in the hospital or is she home? Is she up and about yet?

The messages arrived on our phones, in our email inboxes. I began to update the blog.

Caitlin is not feeling better and is not going to be better until after transplant. Her pulmonary hypertension is severe and contributing to her high oxygen needs. In addition to her nasal cannula, she wears a mask that simultaneously delivers extra, high-flow oxygen. It is hard for her to do anything, as she gets breathless and quickly loses oxygen saturation in her blood. She needs help to do basic things, to move from the bed to the chair, or to shower. A shower is a half-hour, 2-person effort. And a wheelchair ride off the floor, which she and I did alone and fairly easily 2 weeks ago, when she was first admitted, had to be done very slowly yesterday, with four oxygen tanks and her nurse accompanying us.

My posts were a dispassionate cover for heartbreak, for the way it felt to bring Henry in for a visit and see the joy on her face as she hugged the little guy. For the anguish I felt when I handed her a soapy washcloth, rubbed shampoo into her scalp, helped her towel-dry her body, arms, back, down each leg, like when she was a child.

But Heather was just one floor down, her recovery hard but uphill. And Amanda, too, was recovering on a floor somewhere nearby.

And offers were coming in for Caitlin. It was just that the donors were always too large, too old, too *something*.

❦

During those final days of November in that Christmas-lit room at the end of the hall, much that felt surreal and magical began to happen. Birds hovered outside the window. Caitlin began talking in an unfiltered, open, and wise way, about life, to those she came in contact with. At the same time she experienced what she called "weird creative urges." One day she asked for scissors and crayons. Drawing and cutting and filling in her creation with blue pigment was an exhaustive effort that took two days, but she used materials at hand—children's crayons and a plastic medicine cup and a tiny ceramic Virgin Mary to create an exquisite little three-dimensional piece of art.

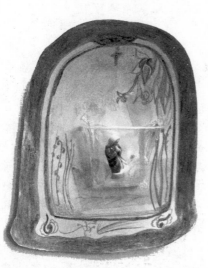

One night a man named Patrick reached out to me via email. He had discovered our blog while researching my novel and felt drawn to connect with our family for reasons he outlined in a long letter that included poetry and encouragement and his sharing of the fact that he and his wife had recently lost a son to cancer.

But here was the wild thing: Patrick was a scientist and patented coinventor of Kalydeco, the Vertex Pharmaceuticals miracle drug that had come, bittersweetly, too late for Caitlin. His random missive in the midst of our situation seemed—surreal. Lovely. I read his words to Nick and Caitlin and it offered us strange strength, as if it were reassurance from the universe.

Back at our apartment that night, I closed my eyes and told myself that all would turn out well. I had just started to nod off when an image of a big white bird flapping straight toward my face made me sit bolt upright in the dark.

⟡

11/28/2016

CAITLIN: I miss you. Sorry I've been so quiet.

JESS: Caitlin E. O'Hara. Can you please never say sorry to me again? I understand your quiet.

CAITLIN: I feel so horrible plus so PMS. I just closed my eyes and envisioned myself in a giant pool of chocolate and then scratching people's eyes out, screaming down the street.

JESS: Ah, little buddy. How are you holding up?

CAITLIN: Up and down. Practicing patience.

JESS: I wasn't going to go but I am leaving for India tonight. 10 days. I am taking you with me.

CAITLIN: Please take me with you. I would so love to go there.

JESS: I know. I'm going for both of us.

CAITLIN: I am going to hope I get transplanted.

JESS: You will be in my backpack. I'm going to come see you when I am back.

CAITLIN: Will you visit someplace spiritual for me?

JESS: Of course.

CAITLIN: By yourself.

JESS: Promise.

CAITLIN: Where are you going?

JESS: Delhi, Coimbatore, Udaipur, Jaipur & Agra

CAITLIN: How are you doing

JESS: I am okay. I think about you so very much. So much. I can't even explain it.

CAITLIN: Thank you.

JESS: I haven't told anyone that I am going to India because everyone feels the need to express their opinion on what I should and shouldn't do so I have just been quiet lately and doing my own thing.

CAITLIN: That's great. People's opinions lead you astray.

JESS: Yes. I learned that from you. ♥

CAITLIN: :) Sometimes they are needed but with a grain of salt. I hate the feeling of having lost my inner guidance because I asked for too much advice.

JESS: How are you feeling emotionally?

CAITLIN: I am just visualizing a lot. Praying a lot. Trying to have daily goals and get through each minute.

It's very hard.

I feel so sick.

December began on a Thursday that year. I see that. The calendar says so. I frantically search my text messages and datebooks and piece together what happened when and how, as if I might be able to rearrange the past and change it. Could we have changed the outcome? We did not expect that stability could collapse like cardboard.

Andrew went back to Maine for the weekend, which seems

like a crazy idea now, but at the time made sense. He would deal with bills and tenants and maintenance at his house, then return on Monday and stay in Pittsburgh indefinitely. If she were to be called over the weekend, he could fly back right away.

Friday night was the first night she would sleep alone in the hospital. She asked me to stay.

"Oh, bud . . ." The days were so long and hard that I looked forward to regrouping each night at home before getting up and starting all over again. Also, I can bear anything if I get my sleep. If I don't, I am no good to anyone. And we needed me during the day.

"You'll be fine," I argued. I would stay until bedtime and promised I would be back first thing.

At the apartment, I prepped ingredients for her lunch: a bone-broth chicken soup. Then I texted her to make sure she was okay before we went to sleep. I told her I was planning to put up a blog post the next day and did she want to add anything? She did and sent it along.

MARYANNE: that's good stuff bud.

CAITLIN: So add to the blog?

MARYANNE: ok

CAITLIN: Thanks. I had to say something
I don't think it's very good but I don't care

MARYANNE: i like it. it's stream of consciousness.

CAITLIN: I need people to know what's going on
Is it awful to want people to pray for you

MARYANNE: NO
of course not. what else is life for but to look out for people

CAITLIN: Ok
I feel like I am begging
For anything. For relief

MARYANNE: i know.

i think there's only one way out and that's through it. let's pray it happens sooner rather than later.

CAITLIN: Ok

I am scared of the night

What was wrong with me? Why didn't I run right back into the hospital? I put up a blog post and let her stay alone in that room, scared of the night.

※

9LivesNotes Post: 12/3/2016

Caitlin: "Answers to ?s"

I love my mummy for everything she does—there are no words. Nor for Andrew and my dad. They are all so caring. focused their lives directly on me. it is hard to reconcile how that can possibly be ok. But I guess it's what we do as humans.

Heart and humor, and humility he said will lighten up your heavy load. Joni Mitchell refuge of the roads.

So much outpouring of love and attention makes humility a challenge, but I am so grateful for it. Heart and humor are easier. They feel like the only directions to go right now. Joni Mitchell's words feel like permission to let go.

I do realize that not everyone who reads this blog is experiencing a big emotional moment in their lives . . . that sometimes life skates around on top where things are delightful and easy. And I've been there and hope to be back, even though I love to cry (with happiness!).

I couldn't be further from the road right now in Joni's song with its literal talk about the refuge of anonymity, cold water restrooms and a photograph of the earth in a highway service station. I am consumed with myself and it's boring and uncomfortable and embarrassing to have so much attention. And I LIKE attention. At the same time I can't stop—in order to keep going I have to focus on myself. Self self self. It feels so anti-human. It is. I rely on others completely and ultimately, finally will rely on another person to keep me alive.

My thoughts these days aren't the skate-on-top kind of normal life thoughts. They're up and down and trippy and depressive— and we have a lot of laughs. And lots of crying. And weird creative urges. I just want to say thank you for listening to what sometimes must be very emotionally over the top sounding writing. And to reassure you I don't take myself too seriously. I do take life seriously though, I'll be honest . . . because it's a seriously wild business.

Thank you for the support—I know I wouldn't survive at all without it. It's such an easy thing to say. But truly, I'd be dead by now! I am so very grateful even if I am a bit off the grid lately and I've faltered shamefully in my thank you notes—I don't think I'll ever get to some of them. But—I'm here, and thank you. And I love everyone very much and love hearing from people even if I am not able to write back.

12/3/2016

1:51 a.m.

CAITLIN: I've been ignored all night. Everyone here tonight is mean. I've had horrible anxiety

CAITLIN: And I've told everyone. Been very vocal about my needs

CAITLIN: And I fell asleep and woke up with sat at 99 and horrible headache. No fluids started still.

CAITLIN: Went to bathroom and couldn't breathe. Was pressing call button and she just keeps saying can I help you I can't hear you. My nurse comes in finally. Literally no one else around tries to help

CAITLIN: I am not nice. Tell her what I think but I'm shaking

CAITLIN: She's like I know sorry I've just been busy. I said well that's why I asked both you and the RT to check on my sats

CAITLIN: I seriously would have been better at home with what just happened

CAITLIN: Oh and as I was having the attack I wasn't on the monitor and I'm shaking to get myself back on bc I think I'm going to pass out

4:43 a.m.

MARYANNE: Buddy! Not sure why I'm not hearing the chime!

CAITLIN: This is pure torture

CAITLIN: It's like hours and hours of hyperventilating. Can't breathe.

CAITLIN: No one helping

CAITLIN: I love you. Send reiki. Trying to sleep.

MARYANNE: Daddy is on his way in.

❦

I arrived at the hospital with food and a nutritional shake and the nasal rinses I prepared each day. Nick had complained to the head nurse, but Caitlin had put the night behind her, and begged us to do so, too. She needed to use her limited energy to recover, move on.

But it was Saturday. And it was the worst kind of hospital weekend, the kind I had dreaded all her life: a weekend crew made up of part-time staff we did not know.

To control her rising CO_2 levels, the team on duty wanted to put her on the bipap machine—basically noninvasive ventilation—which she disliked and had never tolerated. While she was hooked up to it, the mask covering her face, she could not speak and closed her eyes.

❧

I still can't look at the photograph for more than a single gut punch of a second. It was there when I opened my phone and glanced at my Facebook feed.

"Save Prouty Garden shared a photo"
We are utterly heartbroken. 💔

The photo showed a giant crane towering over the sacred earth that had been the Prouty Garden, the dawn redwood tree chopped at its roots, its trunk and limbs piled onto a red flatbed truck.

I felt myself pitching forward with fury, filled with grief and blind anger, and deep, deep despair.

I glanced at Caitlin's face behind the bipap mask and prayed that no one would tell her about it. She was the only focus now.

After the bipap session, she said she felt worse and spent the day having many conversations with the attending and others who came in and out, juggling her situation as only she, the maestro of her body, could do. She said she wanted to be moved to the MICU. The attending on duty did not think it necessary and suggested more bipap sessions. Even I shot down the MICU idea. A move to an ICU seemed intense, unnecessary, stressful.

She knew best, of course.

Late in the afternoon, as she did every night now, she asked for Reiki. This time she physically grabbed my right hand and pressed it hard against her abdomen. "We're connected," she said, her eyes filling with tears. "I'm sorry."

"Sorry for what, bud? Don't be silly. I love you."

A little later she said it. "They cut down the tree."

She was focusing inward, revealing no emotion, and I raged inwardly, too, at the people who had ordered the cutting of the beautiful old tree, knowing its power as symbol, and I raged at this timing, when her health was so vulnerable. Maybe I should have said something about magical thinking. *If you tied the survival of that tree to your own survival, please don't!* I might have said.

Instead I replied that yes, I'd heard, and that karma would come for the people responsible, and that we couldn't think about it right now. Right now we had to be positive and focus on her.

She said okay. She said she might need help in the night and that I shouldn't plan on getting much sleep.

I slipped home to get more food and to gather my overnight supplies. I would be back within the hour, I said, and on my way back, she texted.

CAITLIN: I do not feel right. I'm getting worse and worse
MARYANNE: I'm on my way.
CAITLIN: I don't want to do anything that will put me into
respiratory overdrive
So very slow movements. Bare minimum. Can't get short of breath.
MARYANNE: Walking in right now bud.

She slept poorly and in the morning could barely move. She forced down a few spoonfuls of yogurt. Only then, with almost three years to prepare for this, did I think to ask for her phone password, and where I might find the account information for her monthly bills.

She slept. She slept all afternoon. To Nick and me, it seemed she was catching up on the sleep she had not received the previous two nights. But at about 8:00 p.m., the pulmonologist on duty explained that they could not get her plummeting sodium or elevated CO_2 under control. They were moving her to the MICU, where she could get better care. We were to stay in the family waiting room until they stabilized her.

We waited. And waited. I was mainly confused. I finally rang the nurses' station and they said it was still going to be a while. I asked to come in, I said that Caitlin would want me there. They said no.

Late in the evening, Nick saw staff rushing to the MICU. Then, at about midnight, Dr. Hayanga summoned us into a conference room. He spoke gravely and urgently, explaining ECMO and that they needed our permission to put her on it, that it was necessary to save her life. He handed us pens, forms. We had to sign. *Now.*

We signed like robots and he gathered the papers, ready to bolt. "She won't remember any of this," he said, and added that the good thing was, her score would be as high as it possibly could be, in the 90s. She was now at the top of the list at UPMC, and her high score made her a national priority, too.

We found an empty family room with two reclining chair-beds. We were going to need our sleep, and we tried, our coats thrown over us like blankets, but when we closed our eyes it was all dark terror.

Then bright, eye-biting light: a stumbling, lost-looking couple who recognized themselves in our own faces and quickly snapped off the light, backed out of the room.

Focus: Heather had been on ECMO. Amanda had been on ECMO. Both of them in this very same hospital, just weeks ago. They were breathing with new lungs. And there had been Caitlin's Boston CF friend Meg and her own month-long coma after transplant. And the man from our orientation back in 2010. And a stranger who read our blog and had written to say she'd been in a medically induced coma, her family told she was too sick to transplant, and now she was transplanted and doing well and Dr. D'Cunha had been her surgeon.

Focus: Caitlin was a national priority now. She was first on the list. We had to hold tight. Hold tight. Hold hope tight.

At 3:00 a.m., a nurse from the MICU called. They were moving her down to the CTICU on the third floor. We could see her there.

11

"HOPE" IS THE THING WITH FEATHERS

"Hope" Is the Thing with Feathers

"Hope" is the thing with feathers—
That perches in the soul—
And sings the tune without the words—
And never stops—at all—

And sweetest—in the Gale—is heard—
And sore must be the storm—
That could abash the little Bird
That kept so many warm—
I've heard it in the chillest land—

And on the strangest Sea—
Yet—never—in Extremity,
It asked a crumb—of me.

—EMILY DICKINSON

We buzz into the ICU and put on gowns, gloves, masks. There is a crowd around the bed in the first bay to the right. She is in the same bay where we waited through the dry run just ten days ago.

The crowd parts and I see her, lying rigidly, neck arranged on two flat pillows. Her eyes latch onto the sight of me.

I expected her to be unconscious. Unconsciousness is easier to witness, easier to bear. Inserted into her neck is a garden-hose-size cannula, red with blood.

Inside, I am fainting with fright. My hands grip the bedrails. I lean over them the way I leaned over her crib, and kiss her forehead through my paper mask. "We've been right here, buddy. We love you. We love you so much. It's going to be okay."

"I remember everything." She speaks quietly but fiercely. "They told me I wouldn't remember but I remember everything."

I try to assess the ECMO setup without revealing my horror. Another cannula has been inserted into her groin. The cannulas circulate her blood and connect to a piece of monitoring equipment at the foot of the bed. She is nearly immobile, able only to move her arms.

Her nurse is making adjustments, and when he steps outside the bay, she says, "He's not nice. Trust me. *Trust me.*

"You guys need to watch everything, question everything. *Everything.*

"Promise me you won't leave me. *Promise.*"

Then she points one finger at a woman who is standing to one side quietly observing, clearly monitoring everything that is going on in the bay. "You're good," she says.

The woman introduces herself as Penny Sappington, the medical director of the CTICU. She tells us that she had been part of the team that performed the ECMO procedure up in the MICU, and as she talks I see that Penny is the best kind of doctor: smart and steady, someone you can trust to speak with clarity, empathy, and honesty.

With ECMO, various factors—oxygenation, flow rates, coagulation—must be constantly monitored and fine-tuned. Even so, it's not possible to duplicate the miracle that is the human body's maintenance of health, especially when one major organ has failed and another, in this case, the heart, has been harmed by the other's failure.

During the procedure Caitlin's heart went into SVT three times. She had to be shocked five times. "Her heart is very very sick," Penny says. But she adds that pressure on the heart will reverse with transplant.

Penny casts an appraising, admiring look Caitlin's way and tells me, as she often will in the coming days, "As soon as I saw her, I said to myself, there's something about that girl."

⁂

Morning. The ICU humming quietly. Nick gone to empty the room on the tenth floor—the room that had filled so quickly with the refrigerator and Christmas tree and photographs and suitcases.

At the 7:00 a.m. shift change, a young nurse enters the bay with the kind of skilled, capable self-possession that can't be faked, and I'm relieved. Caitlin will be in good hands for the next twelve hours. She approaches the bed, looks Caitlin in the eyes, and says, "Hi, Caitlin. I'm Erin and I'm going to be your nurse today."

Erin and Caitlin connect immediately. They talk about God and faith, and when Erin steps out of the bay, Caitlin asks me to please do a blog post. "Need prayers. Need ferocious positivity from everyone."

I write a quick post, and afterward, messages flood my email and phone and Facebook account. I sit near the head of her bed, trying to read them aloud, but my voice keeps breaking. My throat is all pain. She worked so hard, tried so hard. She can't move, can't turn her head, make herself comfortable, can't reach an itch. She normally chugs water all day but now can only suck on a damp sponge or risk aspirating. It's like a horror movie; it's like *The Diving Bell and the Butterfly*, the story that had long terrified her.

"It's okay to cry, Mummy." She starts to cry, too.

"I love you so much," she says. "I've never loved anyone as much as you. You've been so good to me my whole life."

It's starkly clear that a complicated medical situation is best overseen by one person who knows and understands absolutely everything. That one person is Caitlin, has long been her, and really, at this late date, can only be her. As good as everyone else is, no one can know everything. Only she does, and she's panicking and she turns to Nick, who is accustomed to running projects and organizing people, and who, unlike me, can function on little sleep. He calms her, and reminds her that we are keeping her stable so that she will get lungs and that he will watch everything, question everything.

Even so, she begins to try to do everything she can to control her situation. She asks for paper and pen, and I give her my new journaling notebook. All day, she writes nonstop: checklists, questions to ask the surgeons, items for Dr. Pilewski.

She pulls no punches. When a resident or technician does something wrong: "You should have known. Don't do it again." "I usually say please and thank you but I can't waste the breath." To a resident who starts to examine her: "You just touched your hair. Change your glove."

To the nurse on the night shift: "You're good. I bet you're a Capricorn."

"I am," he says and smiles.

"I bet you're good with money."

"I would be if I had some."

But she isn't letting herself sleep and is speaking in a flat, blunt, odd way, and that is beginning to alarm me. I reason that she has been through a lot, that after sleep, she will come back to herself. She does not sleep. Instead, she becomes increasingly hard to communicate with and does not stop talking. She writes in the notebook with a frantic intensity—ideas, new plans, instructions for all of us, lists, trying to account for every contingency, every potential issue. Her heart goes into SVT again, and she has to be paddle-shocked. I stay in the bay while they do it but I face the wall and squeeze my eyes shut, stop up my ears. I scream inside my head.

Still, she does not sleep. By 4:00 a.m., more than twenty-four hours after she entered the CTICU, she is no longer making sense.

It isn't even like she is Caitlin.

I learn that sleep deprivation on top of trauma is common in the ICU and has a name: ICU psychosis.

Andrew returns from Maine to stagger, blinking, into this new reality.

And Jess is on her way. She will fly from India to San Francisco for chemo, then fly straight to Pittsburgh.

⁂

SINÉAD: I feel a sense of panic from her. Completely overwhelmed. She's afraid not to be in control. I also feel an ache in the right leg. At the groin area. It's an odd sensation that I can't put into words. Her fear is making her seem angry. Does that make sense? But it's not anger I'm picking up . . .

MARYANNE: She is terrified.

SINÉAD: I'm very aware of her hands. Especially the left? I've never felt her anxiety like this before . . . I'm going to see what they can tell me. Two seconds.

MARYANNE: Let me explain. She can only move her arms and her left leg. Her left hand is constantly holding a suction thing. She can only lie rather flat so it's hard to cough up secretions. When she does, she uses the suction thing to get them out.

MARYANNE: She's got a big catheter in her groin. Also a large garden hose sized one in her neck. The blood goes out of her body, into the "lung machine" and back into her body.

SINÉAD: Ok why can't she move her right leg? It feels like there's a watery sensation in her right leg . . .

MARYANNE: The right leg had the catheter first. It's swollen.

SINÉAD: It's terrifying. She's being so hard on herself. She needs to trust the doctors. I feel like there's a lack of trust.

I am home for a shower during this text exchange with Sinéad, and about to head back to the hospital when Nick calls and tells me to stay put. Caitlin still hasn't slept, he says, and is still writing as fast as she can in the notebook. The team thinks it best that we not see her for a while.

He puts me on to Penny, who says that she is no longer stable and that the team has decided to intubate her. Intubation will allow her to breathe on a ventilator to rest her body and her lungs. She's having trouble coughing, so tomorrow the team will also do a bronchoscopy, a form of cleaning out the lungs. None of this is ideal, but it's not uncommon and now necessary. I ask, "Has she settled down at all?" Penny says, "No, she is scribbling away, never saw a person write so fast."

I stay at the apartment, too stiff with fear to do anything but hold Henry and wait for word. When Erin calls to say that Caitlin is finally sleeping, she tells me about how out of control and combative Caitlin had become. Thrashing, panicky. "Right before sedation, I told her, 'Caitlin, I don't care what you say or do. Right now, I'm going to save your life.'" And that seemed to get through to her. On the vent, Erin says, she can be a bit more sedated, and as comfortable as possible, until transplant.

I look at the audibly ticking clock on my desk, the one Caitlin gave me last Christmas. The hands. They keep moving, relentless. Nick texts, *Try and get some rest.*

I try. I lie down and close my eyes and when I do, the white bird flies at my face, wings spread.

I sit up. What is that? Why is that happening?

Sleep is impossible.

When I return to the ICU, Heather's sister stops by our bay and tells me of Heather's ECMO experience, her equally frightening ICU psychosis.

And up in the cafeteria I run into Amanda and her mother. They tell me that this is Amanda's first time on her feet since her transplant. Amanda, who had been on ECMO and intubated and trached and had been on dialysis.

Now, three and a half weeks after living through this identical trauma, to see her moving and breathing independently is almost biblical, a kind of miracle, like seeing Lazarus.

They were dates on a calendar, two weeks in December. But to live inside those days was to live inside another dimension.

There was constant monitoring to ensure detection of the pulses in her feet, a trip to the OR when they could no longer detect them in the left, swollen leg, site of the arterial cannula. We learned a new word, *fasciotomy*—long cuts to the fascia on either side of her calf to release the pressure.

We adapted to each piece of terrifying news. *Scars. She can live with scars.*

Time bled into another day and another day after that and now she's mostly sedated, but sometimes she swims up to consciousness, and when she does, she's agitated and alert. She fights, digs her nails into us, tries to shout. At one point she points to the breathing tube in her mouth, then makes a writing motion.

Andrew grabs her white board, which he had propped up where she could see it with the words he'd written: *Hi Caitlin. We love you.*

She scrawls one word. *Transplanted?*

No one wants to say no. We say "not yet." We say "soon."

She begins to write more, faster and faster. It is hard to make out all the words, but there are clearly angry ones: "Mistake." "Fucked up."

Her oxygen levels go down with her agitation so we wrestle the white board away, encourage her to close her eyes, relax, give her hand massages, play her *Inspiration 1* playlist. *Under pressure . . .*

⸙

Nick receives an urgent text, then a call from a friend in Massachusetts. He takes the call outside in the corridor, and when he returns, his eyes are full of tears and his voice is breaking with emotion. The friend's wife's cousin has just died unexpectedly in Maine. She was only in her thirties, and petite, like Caitlin. She had O+ blood. The family wants to do a direct donation.

We force ourselves to remain calm. Nick gives Penny the contact information, and Penny, in her measured way, says okay, she will look into it.

Transplantation involves a lengthy set of procedures that take time. The donor lungs have to be assessed several times, at the donor site, for the initial "looks good, let's continue" go-ahead. When the UPMC transplant team gets that okay, two surgical fellows fly to the donor location to do the rest of the tests that will determine if an offer is viable.

It's evening and we are standing by Caitlin's bed when Penny approaches and says that two surgeons are on their way to Maine. With her is Dr. Shigemura, one of the UPMC team's most skilled surgeons, whom Penny has asked to do the surgery. Now she lets herself smile, and hugs us all. She has been orchestrating this all day, but didn't want to get our hopes up until it was a go.

There is such joy, then. Such relief. And humility and gratitude. And *Maine*. It feels so right. So complicated and painful and beautiful and *right*.

Soon Larry, the transplant coordinator for Mallory and Amanda, joins us. He says that Caitlin's regular coordinator is off and he will be acting as the coordinator for this offer. Neither Nick nor I has seen or heard from Caitlin's coordinator and we like Larry. He is compassionate and knowledgeable and Nick asks him to please become Caitlin's permanent coordinator.

We won't really know anything until morning, but we imagine the small plane making its way to Maine, the grief that needed to happen in one family for joy to happen in ours. Caitlin struggled with this—with the fact that her need to live depended on another person's death. She wasn't sure it was right, even though it made practical sense, and she had agreed to it. "There is no reconciling the trade, of life for life, and no justifying it," she once wrote.

And now, the little voice in the back of my mind remembers the psychic who'd thumped her chest and told Katie, "Good match. Accident."

I ask Nick to find out how the cousin passed. She was so young, it had to have been an accident.

He reports back. It was an aneurysm.

Stop, I tell myself. *Stop the superstition.*

But the knowledge tempers my hope, as much as I try to ignore it and focus on the ferocious positivity Caitlin has asked for.

In the morning, we are all on standby in her bay—nurses, fellows, residents, anesthesiologists in place around her bed. We wait for word. I stand close to Caitlin's ear. She's barely conscious but I know she will hear me when I whisper, *It's a go! They have lungs for you!*

The doors to the ICU swing open and Dr. Shigemura walks in, looking troubled, almost vexed. The woman had been a heavy smoker, and young as she was, her lungs were in such ravaged condition, they could not be used.

⁂

MARYANNE: 2nd no go. I love you so much. I miss my buddy.
I love you.
MARYANNE: I love you so much.
I can't live without you.
Please stay stable so we can get a donor for you.
Keep calm in there. Go deep inside. Go somewhere else for a while and let your body remain calm and stable and ready for surgery.

MARYANNE: Caitlin, I'm sitting beside your bed and my throat is full trying to be brave for you. I love you so much, it kills me to see you like this. I can't believe that 3 nights ago you were talking and writing a mile a minute, amusing the staff here. And now you're sedated, and hooked up to every cannula and IV and monitor possible. I am praying that you stay stable and that a donor comes through. I went for a walk on the bridge and my heart was breaking to be there without you. I could hardly look at the photographs, but I wanted to see the yaks and when I got over to that side, where the pine trees are, I saw it was snowing. I've felt your transplant would be in winter, and snow is winter. Oh my bud. I love you more than anything else in this world.

The *knowing* was happening, I can admit that now. Something felt *stuck*, no matter how desperately I wanted to will a transplant to happen quickly.

At the same time, "four" began to show up, in weird ways. Four-leaf clovers began to show up, the most notable being a small, green plastic one that appeared at my feet one day when I ran home to take Henry out.

She'd been on ECMO four days when the surgeons performed a tracheostomy, an opening in the windpipe that would allow easy access between her body and the ventilator, as well as access to her airways. It got the breathing tube out of her mouth, made her more comfortable, and helped her oxygenation.

Dr. D'Cunha talked to us at her bedside and to assure Caitlin, who was briefly conscious, that all had gone well. "We'll get you transplanted this weekend, Caitlin," he said.

Okay, I thought. *He's saying the words. It will happen.* I tried to convince myself even though I knew that there was no way he could be certain, that he was just projecting positivity.

Then he turned away to remove his mask, gown, and gloves for disposal. He bent over to wash his hands and as he straightened, I saw him hesitate. I sensed that his glance had landed on a particular photograph—of Caitlin and Jess, out in the city one summer night: young and beautiful and beaming.

And his shoulders slumped.

He was only human, too.

We accompanied him out of the ICU and into the hall, where we could talk more freely. She was already in better overall condition because of the trach, he said, but he sighed, too. "I'll feel a lot better when this one's transplanted, though."

Nick asked, "Anything?"

"No. But I have a good feeling about this weekend."

I was desperate. I grabbed at those words. *Really? Okay. Good.* They must mean *something.* "Okay," I said uncertainly.

"She's the sickest person in the United States," he said. "She's the sickest person who needs a lung transplant in the United States. You can quote me."

<hr />

The days seemed longer than they were. They seemed to stretch out, and Penny was always there and Erin couldn't have always been on duty but it seemed she was. She washed and braided Caitlin's hair and the three of us took turns so that someone was always by Caitlin's side.

I wrote blog posts to update people and for the first time revealed my desperation. I wrote about direct donations, a wonderful thing in a terrible time. I outright begged:

Caitlin O'Hara is 5' 2" and has a blood type of O+ and is on life support at UPMC, Pittsburgh.

She received a third offer of lungs. Dr. D'Cunha seemed optimistic and confident but reminded us that initial assessments were based on CT scans and blood gases. Outside indicators.

We knew. And we knew the routine by now: *Try to sleep. Count the hours until morning. Stand by her bed, wait for the yes,* but again, the offer was a no-go.

In this case, the left lower lobe had been damaged by pneumonia. A strange coincidence, since Caitlin's left lower lobe was the one that had been damaged and removed when she was eleven.

It's been snowing all morning. Christmas carols play in the public spaces. Caitlin's bay is cozy, glowing with the Christmas lights we hung behind her bed, and with the wall of photographs of normalcy. Family. Friends. Home. Henry.

She is unconscious nearly all the time now, but we constantly tell her how much we love her. And that Jess will arrive soon. *On Tuesday! Your buddy will be here.*

I put on the playlists she'd asked me to create back in September. I hold her hand and tell her things—mainly that her only job now is to stay calm and be strong and trust that we're taking care of her. *Anam Cara,* I tell her, over and over. *You are my soul friend.*

As I talk, I look up at the ceiling and wonder if, like the stories you hear, some part of her consciousness is up there hovering, aware of all that we say and do.

Maybe she is scolding me for playing "Refuge of the Roads" too many times, telling me I am ruining its powers.

But probably she is saying, *It's okay.*

⁂

Two o'clock on Monday morning marks a full week on ECMO, and days of OR ins and outs for all kinds of tinkering. A week is too long to be on ECMO. I ask Dr. D'Cunha if he is tracking any offers. He shakes his head, says he hasn't had one in twelve hours, and those offers were unsuitable, from big men, chests with lungs too large for Caitlin.

My posts become ever desperate. Joe Pilewski is away at a conference, and in twenty-four hours Penny will be leaving for a weeklong one in New York. I'm feeling terrified, adrift.

I write a post about regional allocation injustice and how someone with a score of 40, comfortably waiting at home, in one region, could legally be transplanted over Caitlin because regions have first dibs on their region's donors. I appeal again for direct donation awareness.

And I become vaguely aware that a kind of big swell begins to happen. Friends, acquaintances, old and new connections, people getting in touch with other people, contacting us with ideas. Writers are writing. Talkers are talking. Reporters are reporting. An offer comes from the Philippines—too far away. A woman from our Pittsburgh apartment building loses a family member, and the family makes Caitlin the offer, but the donor is too tall. Julian Edelman tweets about Caitlin. A PR friend in New York arranges for me to talk to *People* magazine. The head of a busy transplant center in Baltimore, which has newly begun to transplant people with cepacia, in that city with its much larger donor pool, is going to drive up to talk to us, see how he can help. Larry has been in constant touch and suggests that we let the Center for Organ Recovery and Education (CORE) publish a feature about Caitlin.

At one point, I log onto the blog and see that it's had sixty thousand visitors in just the past two hours.

Jess has flown in from San Francisco, and Nick has gone to pick her up. I leave Andrew with Caitlin and take my coffee to the top floor of the hospital, into an empty family room where I can stand at the window and look down on the city and the large, leafy park beyond the university. As I sip my coffee, a hawk glides by the window, so close that I think, *Okay, something is going on with birds! I need to record this.*

I leave myself a voice message. I say, "It's like we had to be kicked in the face to really appreciate this life. Even after all these years with CF." I say, "Tonight is the third and final supermoon of the year. It's called the Cold Moon." I say, "I feel like I've gotten some kind of calling. I keep getting that message, 'Help people into the next life.' I guess this story can help people and give them courage so I am going to have to tell it." I say, "People want to believe."

Then I return to the ICU, where Andrew is holding one of Caitlin's hands and Caitlin is unconscious, looking like she can never be conscious again. I remind myself that Amanda looked like this, Heather looked like this, Meg was in a coma, and on and on.

I am due to talk to *People* magazine in two hours.

I bend over Caitlin to kiss her forehead and glance up, hope flaring at the sight of Dr. D'Cunha walking through the ICU doors, heading toward us.

But his face is not the face of a surgeon with an offer. "Can we speak privately?" he asks.

Andrew and I look at each other as we follow him out of the ICU and into a quiet hallway, and my fear is a fast-beating heart and a mind racing *what-what-what-what-what*.

He takes a breath and says it: that he's so sorry, that she's become too sick to transplant, that it is probably time to gather family around.

I have a memory of such mental crumpling that I am not sure what my body did but I found myself near the floor, Andrew there with me, and everything is *no, no, no*. This is the same man whose words, just days earlier, were, "We'll get you transplanted, Caitlin."

No. I get to my feet. I refuse to believe that this is it. That after all this time and struggle, she isn't even going to get a chance. I focus on one fact: "Is there any hope at all that she can improve enough to be transplanted?"

Any improvement would be a long shot, he says.

A long shot is still a shot. She still has a shot. And Caitlin has always beaten the odds. Caitlin O'Hara has nine lives.

Next I remember I am by her bed, kissing her head, whispering, *Buddy, buddy, I love you we have to get you well.*

But there is such despair, such weary, defeating despair. Such backtracking. Now she is not even on the list.

And Penny is leaving, due to teach at that conference in New York.

I call Nick and tell him and he's like me, gut-punched but scrambling—how can we still make this work? I ask my brother to cancel the *People* magazine interview. I am incapable of talking, and also, how can I announce that she is no longer listed? I can't tell people. The hope and prayers and energy and awareness—they're all too strong and powerful. We still need that hope, need those prayers.

Nick arrives with Jess beside him. She is clutching his arm, walking stiff and upright, her face a mask of shock. Once inside the ICU bay, she takes Caitlin's hand and speaks in her steady, determined way. "I am never going to leave her side."

Nick tugs on my arm. "Let me take you home. You'll feel better after a shower."

❦

Our condominium is just a short trip away, down a stretch of highway, and as Nick merges onto the ramp, a huge white hawk, wings outstretched, flies straight toward my face, so close I protect my head with my hands, thinking he will hit the windshield.

But he swoops up and over the roof, and Nick and I look at each other, eyes wild. *What was that? What was that we just saw?*

I tell Nick about the white bird images that have come to me these past weeks. "Just as I'm trying to sleep." The same stretched-out wingspan of white feathers, the sharp eyes and beak, the flapping straight toward my face.

We both agree: it had to be a sign . . . right?

And when we return to the hospital, there is Penny in the ICU. I ask what she is still doing here. Isn't she going to New York?

She shakes her head, says she canceled her appearance at the conference, and I am so overcome with gratitude and love for this woman that I want to weep.

Her monitoring presence becomes constant. Once, in the middle of the night, I even find her asleep in a chair by Caitlin's bay.

The surreal quality of the next few days. The intensity. The vigilance. Sleeping in the family room chairs in the corner we claim as our own. Taking turns by Caitlin's bed, Jess giving her three-hour hand massages, Andrew writing long letters for Caitlin to read later, me playing her musical playlists, reading aloud from Mary Oliver's new *Upstream*, which weirdly but beneficially always improves her blood pressure. The cocoon of Christmas lights and religious gifts hanging from her IV poles—a crucifix, a Star of David, a Celtic cross, a rosary—the nightly delivery of home-cooked meals from the Squirrel Hill community of kind strangers. The friends and family who all want to visit and we say, *No-thank-you-no, we've got some magic going on here*. The Baltimore doctor who visits and says he can definitely get her a donor and is willing to try to move her but she is far too ill to move, and now the broadcast news stories are happening. I briefly see a video of one of them; we have become one of those tear-jerking Christmas stories: a photograph I've never seen of a stunning Caitlin back in 2011 holding a Fourth of July sparkler with the headline FAMILY HOPING FOR A MIRACLE.

After the Boston television stations run the story, someone from Mass General Hospital, right around the corner from her apartment that *has sat empty for two years*, calls Nick and offers to transplant her, but it's too late, too late for reversal of cruel decisions.

After days of silence, I finally update the blog. I illustrate my post with a photograph of two enormous stone angels that were the first things I saw in my Instagram feed that morning and that I saw as yet another good sign.

Clearly, my silence of the past few days has indicated that it has been a time of waxing and waning health and hope. I'm not going to go into all the details, but Caitlin has had a lot of complications and on Tuesday was temporarily considered "not strong enough to undergo surgery."

BUT—in the past 36 hours, she has made some steady and unexpected improvements. The incredible Penny, the critical care physician here, has pulled all kinds of tricks out of her Mary Poppins bag to help her, and Caitlin's deeply gifted intuitive healer cousin, Sinéad, in London, has been working, nonstop, to read Caitlin (it's uncanny how accurate Sinéad is), and send insights and healing. We all feel the prayers and energy coming from all around our buddy. Probably most importantly, deep inside, Caitlin's inner tiger cat stopped resisting and fighting the help and is now calmly fighting to help herself.

Her liver and kidneys were in trouble, and her blood pressure was low. She went on dialysis on Tuesday. By yesterday, they'd cut way back on it, and her body was producing lots of urine on its own, surprising everyone.

She was put on blood pressure support to increase her blood pressure. She's still on blood pressure support meds, but they've been reduced, with no drop in pressure, and that's a good sign. We need for that to continue.

Her liver is still in trouble, but it's a young liver and can bounce back. Still, we need to help it improve, and that means cutting down on the medications she's on.

Her belly was having problems and they've had to stop feeding for a while to give it a break.

So there's a list of stuff to pray for. She's very sick but there is hope. You can read some of the comments on this blog, from other transplant patients, who've "been there and lived to tell the tale."

I'm grateful that strangers have reached out to comfort us with their stories.

The surgeons are still considering all offers for her, but any lungs cannot be less than perfect in her case, they must be Harry Potter lungs. And she must be strong enough to withstand the surgery. So it's a constant monitoring, and a "feel," as her surgeon said.

I cannot thank you all enough for sending so much love and support her way. This has been a difficult emotional time, yet also overwhelmingly uplifting.

Nothing is worth more than love. Nothing.

On Saturday the seventeenth, I notice that Dr. D'Cunha's name has replaced Penny's as Caitlin's doctor on the ICU census board. No one says anything, but I know that the surgeon's name replaces the medical director's name when someone is about to be, or has been, transplanted. Throughout the day, various staff come in and out to perform tests they just say "have been ordered."

That evening, Nick and Andrew and Jess are with Caitlin and I am in the darkened family room about to try and get some rest when my phone rings.

It is Dr. D'Cunha. He tells me he has an offer, a very good offer, and that the entire team agrees that Caitlin deserves this chance, but that it's very, very risky. He needs us to understand that risk. "I can't promise I can bring her through," he says.

I understand, I say. *I understand.* I have never felt such gratitude. I have no doubt that Caitlin can pull through.

All she needed was a chance.

Later that night, I find four pennies on the washbasin. At

1:00 a.m., Larry texts me a photograph of a four-leaf clover key-chain. He writes, *I wouldn't consider myself the most religious person in the world. But I've been praying for the chance to send that to you.*

This offer will be the fourth and can only be the final.

There is a different quality to this offer, I feel it. Less of a sense of wondering whether it will be a go, just knowing that it will be. All we are legally allowed to know is that the donor was young and healthy, but those two facts, I have come to appreciate, are enormous indications of viability.

In the morning they take Caitlin away to the OR early, before we even know if surgery will go forward. We wait and wait, pacing the halls. We are outside the ICU when Dr. D'Cunha's right-hand surgical fellow, Dr. Lara Schaheen, finds us and tells us the lungs are healthy and are on the way to Pittsburgh.

We yelp and hug her. I quickly type a blog post, finally able to post the words I have been desperate to write for three years.

It's a Go.

I am so relieved that I don't have the fear I would normally feel. I put on a Santa hat I'd brought in to cheer Caitlin and that was still in her ICU bay.

I am happy. I am smiling.

We wait in a family room, a quiet one we have to ourselves, on the top floor of the hospital.

At one point I go out into the hall and I'm surprised to bump into Joe Pilewski. He is coming out of the chapel and he is unsmiling and somber. He tempers my joy, telling me that this surgery is a grave risk.

I ask, "But what would you have us do?"

He looks at me as if the answer is obvious. "Let her go to heaven?"

Heaven? Here within these walls of science and medical reason, a doctor I respect and trust is using the word "heaven" and I don't like it and am beginning to be afraid.

I think I say something like "Caitlin will surprise you." I go back to the family room, where we are still holding our collective breath. The organs must arrive safely. It's cold, it's winter. Accidents happen. An accident very likely claimed our donor's life. Once the transplant team views the lungs and Caitlin together, in the operating room, only then will they truly know that they can go ahead.

At 2:44 p.m. I am finally able to post an update.

We got word that the lungs arrived safely to the OR at noon, and just recently got word that the right lung is already in. It was a perfect fit, with no trimming needed. This is what you hope for.

Amanda visits with her mother for a short time. Amanda, who was fighting for her own life just six weeks ago, and has already been discharged. She sits there with a big smile on her face, literally crying with happiness for us.

The mood is good. Buoyant. It lingers through the afternoon. But at about 6:00 p.m., a member of the surgical team comes looking for us. His expression is neutral and he has no "all went well" message. He says only that Dr. D'Cunha needs to talk to us and directs us to a waiting room.

I take off the Santa hat.

In the room, we wait and wait. When Dr. D'Cunha finally comes in, his manner is grave. The transplant is finished, he says; that part of it went well, better than expected.

I take that in. Perfect lungs. An easy transplant. How different everything might have been with an earlier transplant, a healthier and stronger Caitlin.

"But we can't get her off the heart/lung machine," he says. "This is what I was afraid of."

We are all still. Just listening. Barely breathing.

"We'll keep trying." It's all he can say. And then he is gone.

I am desperate again and I phone Sinéad in London, where it is nearly midnight. I ask her if she can tap in, send energy. She does and tells me that Caitlin's energy is still very strong but that something is going on with her left leg, that "it's like pins and needles." That's all she can tell me.

And then a relieved Dr. D'Cunha is back to say they did it, they got her off the heart-lung and back onto ECMO, which they will have to slowly wean her from in the coming days.

She is alive. And she is finally, finally, *finally* on the other side of transplant.

12

ALL THE WORDS

I lived inside blurred moments, that first day after transplant. I wrote sleep-deprived, hyped-up, overly positive posts and used lots of exclamation points, clearly explaining, in detail, the problems Caitlin was facing: her liver and her rising lactate levels, indicative of dead tissue somewhere. *Let's hope they find something that's causing these increasing lactates! This OR trip is proactive and good. Caitlin has a great medical team!*

If there was healing magic in the universe, I wanted every bit of it, every prayer directed toward her specific needs.

I didn't post her photograph, couldn't show the world what those two weeks on ECMO had done to her.

I wrote that my aunt had asked a good question: *Was she aware that she had been transplanted?*

I wrote, *The answer is YES. She's listening. We told her.*

Was she? She must have been. I wrote it. But she would have been barely conscious. She was certainly not communicative. I stood at her bedside, her small face seemingly oblivious to all the cannulas and monitoring wires and alarms, and I wondered where she was.

The miracle transplant had finally happened. Her oxygen saturation was 100 percent. But the rest of her was so battered. If it weren't for the experiences of Amanda and Heather, I would have despaired.

※

Tuesday, December 20

It's early morning and I've taken over from Andrew, who shared watch with Jess before she left for the airport at dawn. She has another round of chemo in San Francisco, but has already texted that she loves us and will be back in a few days for our five-little-pigs Christmas.

All is quiet. I read over Andrew's notes from overnight: *Blood pressure improving. Penny started her on Vitamin K. An EKG showed no seizures but her brain is working slowly at the moment. There is dark discoloration in the fingers on her right hand, caused by lack of profusion during transplant. She will likely lose a fingertip but it's not causing problems right now.*

I stand by her bed and smooth her hair. She's been unconscious most of the past two weeks, but I feel uneasy. Perhaps because of the EKG report, but something feels different now. She doesn't seem to be present.

I look up at the ceiling, wondering, again, if her consciousness is hovering, watching.

Dr. D'Cunha and his team arrive on early-morning rounds. He does not have any special concerns, but tells me that a chest tube on her left side is draining a bit more than he likes. "She's not unstable but I need to take a look. Clean her out."

He tells me he has reserved a standing slot in the OR for the next few days in case he needs to go in like this.

After he moves on, I sit down and open my laptop. I am writing a new blog post about our lucky "four-leaf clover" transplant when the regular CTICU team enters to do their own morning rounds. Penny is finally off-duty and one of the doctors lifts one of Caitlin's eyelids to check her pupils. I see the immediate look of concern, the lifting of the other eye. The quiet commotion. Then the attending, a man named Boujoukos, whom I've not yet met, lifts her lids and shines his penlight into her eyes. I stand up and see for myself the flat gaze, the enlarged pupils. I watch him check her gag reflex. Nothing. He speaks to her with instructions.

Nothing.

O my God, O my God, O my God. No one says a word to me.

I ask.

The doctor is noncommittal, his face a practiced mask. He says they can't assess brain damage or its reversibility until they do a CT scan. But Erin's eyes are red and glassy and I understand why so many ICU nurses burn out early.

~

The terrified waiting. The panic. I've heard that hospitals in some countries have screaming rooms, and I want one. I want to scream, do something with this desperate fear. I call Nick. Text Sinéad, who says she will text me back when she connects. I rest my head next to Caitlin's and whisper over and over, *Please don't go, please don't go.* Nick arrives and urges me to go home and shower and rest and I take the keys and I run like a coward. I want oblivion and to wake from oblivion to the news that everything is all right.

At home, I jump onto my bed and pull a blanket over my head and then throw it off in a panic, sitting bolt upright.

A brain bleed—what she always feared. *I've always thought I was going to die of a stroke.*

I hug Henry. *Oh, Henry Henry Henry I love you so much. Our buddy is sick. Our buddy is so sick.*

SINÉAD: Energy connection wasn't strong. I can feel the following after reading:
—pressure in her head—at the left side mainly at the back
—energy over right ear
—an ache over heart that came and went
—I was still drawn to her abdomen but for healing purposes
—Connection is faint but I'm going to try healing now and see what I can feel/do

Dr. D'Cunha calls, and there's urgency in his voice. He must remove her leg. There is no time to delay.

Dear God. "She can live without a leg," I say. "What about the brain?"

"The leg is more pressing. It has to come first."

SINÉAD: I need to talk to you. Urgent.

I call Sinéad and she speaks quickly, nearly breathless. She says she was trying to energetically connect with Caitlin when the text message window between the two of them popped up on her phone. "I said, 'Okay, Caitlin, what do you have to tell me?' and I got a sudden burst of strong energy across my back, by the scapula on the left side, near the spine."

I am barely conscious of how I get there but I am back at the hospital waiting pacing crying waiting and after the procedure they wheel her to the ICU and I wrap my hands around her knee, kiss the thick bandages. And now they're taking her in for the CT scan and Nick and I go up to the chapel and Andrew is already there and we look at each other and both fall to the floor. Nick tugs on us, *Get up get up we have to be positive*, he is saying.

But I know. I know I know I know I know I know.

I can't pray or breathe or do anything but wait for the horror that's coming for me.

Back down in the family room, I lie on my chair bed and put my coat over my face and stare into the black and Nick comes in and says my name and I stand up and look at him.

It's all there in his broken face, his voice. "I think we're going to lose her," he says.

He holds out his arms and I crumple inside of them.

It all happens so fast then. It all happens so fast.

<hr />

Dr. Boujoukos leads us into a room next to the family room that people use for eating. There are crumbs on the table, someone's crumpled napkin.

He is compassionate and saying all the words but he is also efficient. He explains how he will turn off the ECMO machine. He says she won't feel anything but he can give her something if it makes us feel better.

I ask him to give her Dilaudid.

I expect some time to process what is about to happen, but we sign papers and the doctor rises to his feet and we follow him and it dawns on me that it's going to happen *right now*, and my brain is trying to catch up with my body.

In the ICU bay, my eyes fill up at the battered sight of her.

I stand on her left side by her head, Nick beside me to my left.

Andrew on the opposite side. I slip a copper bracelet sent by her friend Alyssa onto her left wrist. There are words stamped into the metal: BE BRAVE.

We all put our hands on her and I lean into her ear and whisper that it is okay to go, of course it's okay, that I hadn't known how bad everything was earlier, when I begged her to stay.

My eyes flit around the bay. I see that there is a penny on the ECMO machine.

I say yes when Dr. Boujoukos asks if we want the heart monitor on. So many times, in her lifetime of admissions, I have watched that monitor and thanked God that her heart beat and flinched when my mind imagined it otherwise. I feel I must witness the stopping, the line going flat.

And then it is solemn chaos. Dr. Boujoukos doesn't tell us that the ECMO machine beeps horribly in warning when it is unplugged until it is unplugged and he apologizes and says there is nothing that can be done about it.

Erin has closed the curtains to the bay, and Dr. Boujoukos is outside of it but he keeps poking his head in to check and it is a horror show, his face coming through the part in the curtains like *The Shining*.

But it happens very very quickly and there's no stopping time, it's like water running through fingers. The heartline goes flat. The alarms stop.

Penny is on her way in to see us.

Erin asks if we want Caitlin's handprints, if we want to cut some of her hair, the hair that Erin was so careful to wash and braid the past two weeks. We don't expect these questions but don't want to say no and then regret it later, so. Yes.

I smooth her hair and kiss her forehead as the nurses cover each palm with poster paint then press it onto pink construction paper. The result looks like a dozen elementary school art projects I have stored up in our attic.

They snip a thick lock of hair and place it inside a plastic zip bag.

Penny arrives and hugs us and we stand there and say words until it is clear we are not saying anything. But I don't move.

"How can I just walk away?" I ask. "I can't just leave her."

Penny puts one hand over her heart and points upward with the other. "She's not here," she says. She shakes her head, the sorrowful gesture of a doctor who has seen it all.

We back away from the bed and stand at the curtain, looking and looking, taking one more look and then one more. And then another look through the part in the curtains and one more, and this is the last time you will ever see your daughter.

❦

A quick spiral, a death loop, a crash to the ground.

And yet—even though we are numb and stumbling, there is still doing to be done. The niche in the family room we had carved out for ourselves, and which we had expected to stay in for the next few weeks: we have to pack it all up, throw out food, ball up the sheets, say good-bye to the other resident family, people who are solemn and tearful and who hug us good-bye.

Then we are back at the apartment, opening the door on the bittersweet absurdity that is happy, jumping Henry.

Telling Jess. Telling my sister and close friends. They will let everyone else know.

We can't eat. We try to sleep.

At one point in the night I can't take it and throw myself on the floor and scream and scream until I've ripped my throat raw and frightened Henry, who sniffs around my head, whimpering.

Nick helps me up and back to the bed, where I ask the universe to give me an hour of unconsciousness.

Nick and Andrew and I walk over to the Fairmont to get out of the apartment, to get out of our heads. The Fairmont is two blocks, and to get to it, we have to walk through all the holiday goings-on—the ice rink and gingerbread house display signs, the European Holiday Market stalls in Market Square.

On our way back, as we are walking by the ice rink, an urge comes out of nowhere. Let's go see the gingerbread houses, I say. I veer sharply to the right to lead the guys toward the building where they are on display. Along my path, I see a bunch of pennies on the ground. I pick them up, count them.

There are eleven.

I put them in my pocket and walk into the crowded atrium containing the toy trains and glittering displays of gingerbread houses. Standing right in front of me is Kwesi, Teppany's husband, the young man from Trinidad and Tobago who had the lung transplant in 2014. I've only met Kwesi twice before. I know he lives miles from downtown. I can't believe he is right there in front of our eyes and I almost can't speak. But I do and I stammer something about Caitlin and then . . . we leave.

Because I had no real interest in seeing the gingerbread houses. It seemed that I had been shown some things I was supposed to see. The recipient of a successful transplant, and the number eleven, always associated with the year of the lobectomy, the year we might have lost her.

Maybe eleven was a reminder that we had her twenty-two years longer than we might have. And Kwesi, a reminder that we are all on our own paths.

···

A friend of ours has a plane and he sends it to Pittsburgh to bring us home. We Uber to the airfield, where the plane waits with pilots who are respectful and kind.

I buckle Henry into a seat, and the plane is up and then down and it's only two hours since we walked out of the Pittsburgh apartment and now we are in our house. Blinking, disoriented.

Before we left Pittsburgh, we made a quick decision and hastily dismantled Caitlin's little white Christmas tree. Now it glows in the corner by the fireplace, and the cozy loveliness of home is unbearable.

···

The funeral director is urging us to make a decision. People are calling, wanting details.

Once, Caitlin and I had visited the Père Lachaise cemetery in Paris, the famous garden cemetery with its narrow, strollable avenues and ornate mausoleums and Gothic graves. Colette is buried there, and Chopin, and Oscar Wilde and Edith Piaf and Gertrude & Alice and Jim Morrison and pretty much every famous historical Parisian dweller you might imagine. Caitlin was firm the day of that visit. She did not want to be underground. And she definitely did not want cremation. Or a wake or any kind of reception or service in a funeral home.

I tell Nick, "She wanted a mausoleum."

The funeral director tells him that there is a mausoleum and small garden cemetery only three miles away from our home. On the property is a tiny, nonsectarian stone chapel where we can have any kind of service we want. I want to see it.

A friend puts me in her car and I find myself there. The chapel is beautiful in its simplicity: inlaid tile floors; high, cream-colored walls; a soaring ceiling. An arched alcove for an altar, with a blue domed ceiling painted with gold stars and Byzantine sunbeams. Windows made of vitrailed leaded glass with sunburst designs and clear mosaics.

It is aesthetically perfect, and exactly what Caitlin would want, but we can't fit more than a hundred or so people into it, a problem. We have a lot of family, friends, and acquaintances. We have lived in the area for decades. I am hearing that old high school friends of Caitlin's are coming in from everywhere, including someone I've never met, a young woman from Northern California who says that Caitlin was so good to her when her mother died that Caitlin changed her life.

She seems to have affected so many lives.

We finally announce that we will have a small, private service, and something larger later. We'll just have to stuff as many close friends and family as we can into that chapel.

❦

I want the service to be orderly and orchestrated, so I hire a well-regarded officiant. Caitlin's friend Billy offers to do all the printing. He will print four-foot-tall matte portraits of Caitlin, twelve of them, which we will hang between the stained glass windows and in the alcove at the front of the chapel.

I work on the service program, and send photos and music choices to my filmmaker brother Michael for the tribute film.

For the service program book, I include Caitlin's bird artwork, snippets of old texts and emails, and poems and words she lived by—those of Viktor Frankel, W. H. Auden, Virginia Woolf, Leo Tolstoy, Langston Hughes, Primo Levi.

As I work, I remember a trip Caitlin and I made to the Andy Warhol museum in Pittsburgh just a few months earlier. There you could partake in one of Andy's famous "screen tests." The screen test consists of sitting still, unsmiling, and looking straight at a camera, which records you for three minutes, then transforms the finished film clip into four minutes. The result is slowed-down, mesmerizing.

I frantically search my email, sure that Caitlin must have sent me the link for hers. She did, and the screen test still exists, and it's available to download and now it is as if she is there on the other side of my screen, and I am looking into her eyes, connecting with their aliveness. I watch every second of the four minutes, and when I get to the end of it, I realize that it is perfect. The end is perfect. Almost as if she had planned it.

December 30 dawns bright and cold. At one point, a snow squall turns the world angry and white. Then it passes and the air is clear again.

We wait for 3:00 p.m., the time of the service, all of us moving around the house as if we've been shot. What is this? What is this funeral, when we were just living inside the rhythms of the ICU and that was the only reality? What were those hoses in her groin, her neck, all that slicing up of her body? How had that all come to be? I double over with the pain of it, and Nick's face is all pain, too, and Andrew is at our side, and Jess, and I am grateful that Nick and I will not have to walk into that chapel alone like the childless couple we've suddenly become.

As we prepare to leave, I catch sight of myself in a mirror. I think of that astrological reading Caitlin gave me, and how the woman said I was at the start of my "second Saturn return."

A new year. A new life. And no choice in the matter.

⁂

About the mausoleum, Caitlin's friends smile and say, *Only Caitlin!*

Caitlin liked over the top. She liked drama and beauty. As Nick and I walk in flanked by Andrew and Jess, I want this service to celebrate her unique self.

It does. The chapel is like a sacred art gallery, the tall prints lining the walls like fine portraits. Bright afternoon sun streams in through the windows. A friend plays slow-tempo acoustical guitar pieces as we read poetry in unison, and as the hour passes it is as if a sacred spell comes over the space.

Katie approaches the podium first, and then one by one, like an incantation, a stream of Caitlin's close friends follow, each of them poised and articulate and speaking to the strength of Caitlin's character.

Jess struggles at first, then gathers herself and vows to do something extraordinary in Caitlin's name.

Andrew talks about the mountain that Caitlin climbed every single day.

I have arranged for the officiant to take my place if I find myself unable to get up and lead the recitation of "Dogfish," a Mary

Oliver poem Caitlin loved and that I chose for one singular line that called to me.

But I don't need him. I stand at the podium and look out at the crowd a moment. When I begin, my voice surprises me with its strength and I manage to say the line I thought would break me:

*I wanted to hurry into the work of my life; I wanted to know, whoever I was, I was / **alive** for a little while.*

As the service draws to an end, Caitlin's cousin Jillian speaks:

It seems to me that Caitlin came into this world as a great bearer of light. And it also seems to me that her light grew as her health struggles grew. And it seems that her light is now stronger than ever, because it's filling this room. To me, Caitlin more than any other person that I've known, inspires me to live life to the fullest. This is a woman who traveled extensively despite her illness, who brought into her life the kind of deep and loving friendships that have the mark of soul-relationships, who spent her last several years with this incredible man who loved her so deeply and fully, who supported her on her highest path, in her utmost truth. And so, I feel like the gift that Caitlin has brought to us all is the reminder, and even the urging, to live life fully, to not waste a single breath. And if we do waste breath, to not waste more in mourning it, but to forgive ourselves, to forgive others. Kindness and compassion, truth and love, these are what she brought to us as our friend, cousin, niece, daughter, and partner.

My understanding from conversations I've had with Caitlin and also with Maryanne, is that Caitlin was very spiritual, but did not ascribe to any religion. She was more pantheistic. Similarly to how she loved us, she saw and loved the best and what was good, in all religions. I understand that she had always felt an affinity for the Virgin Mary, and I have been asked to lead everyone in a recitation of the Hail Mary prayer in honor of her special connection with the great Mother. As we recite this prayer together now, I invite you to be present with the words as we would be in the reading of a poem, to reflect on the spirit of Mary.

> *Hail Mary,*
> *Full of Grace,*
> *Our Lord is with thee.*
> *Blessed art thou among women,*
> *and blessed is the fruit*
> *of thy womb, Jesus.*
> *Holy Mary,*
> *Mother of God,*
> *pray for us sinners now,*
> *and at the hour of death.*
> *May it be so.*

My brother readies the screen, dims the lights. There is silence. Shuffling. Then the simple rhythmic conga/bongo/snare drum percussions that open Queen's "These Are the Days of Our Lives" fill the chapel.

It is the first time I've seen the film, these scenes of the past coordinated with the heartbreak soundtrack that is Freddie Mercury's voice and lyrics, and for a moment I shake violently and uncontrollably. My brother has fit the images to the music, and there are heartbreaking moments combined with humorous snippets and the entire film is a small feast for our hungry senses.

When it ends, silence crackles, then the four minutes of the black-and-white Andy Warhol screen test begin to roll as Leonard Cohen sings "Hallelujah."

Four long minutes of her eyes looking into our eyes.

I hear the sounds of stifled sobs and quiet crying behind me but I know that as much as Caitlin would want us all to think of her with joy, she very much would also want us to ugly-cry and mourn her. She would revel in the pain and beauty of this service and in this film because she knew, more than anyone, that grief and joy are both points on the spectrum of love.

The screen test rolls on hypnotically, her face unchanging, eyes slowly blinking until close to the final frames, when she abruptly pulls off her oxygen. She maintains eye contact with the camera and allows a brief smile as she twitches her nose and breathes un-aided for another twenty seconds before all fades to white.

Book Three

Afterlife

The great revelation perhaps never did come. Instead
there were little daily miracles, illuminations,
matches struck unexpectedly in the dark.

—VIRGINIA WOOLF

13

"THE REFUGE OF THE ROADS"

12/31/2016

MARYANNE: Where are you?

January 2. A quiet house. Jess on her way back to San Francisco. Andrew finally gone home to Maine.

Nick and I had thought we might go into Caitlin's apartment in Boston but he's not up for it after all, and I'm past functioning. All I can do is flop from one surface to the next and cry.

Andrew sends a picture of a note from Caitlin he found inside his glove compartment when he arrived home. She had jotted down a quote from his favorite childhood story, *Peter Pan*, and signed it with a heart: "To live would be an awfully big adventure."

I imagine her folding the note and slipping it into his car for him to find. *To live*. We all live and we all die and there is nothing in me but doubt and despair and I cry even harder until I cry myself out and end up on the sofa, near her little Christmas tree, and turn on the television, looking to find something we loved, something I can share, and I see that there is, in the DVR folder, a favorite movie we had partly watched this past summer when we were home. *The Remains of the Day.*

We had paused it midpoint and I don't remember why. Were we interrupted, or had it just gotten late, or what? What had actually happened? The amnesia emblematic of all the moments that make up our lives and then are mostly forgotten.

I press RESUME and there is Mr. Stevens on his trip to the west country to try and reclaim all he had lost. "Blue Moon" plays in the 1950s background, and it is all too much, the atmosphere thick with poignancy and regret and our human inability to change the past and then its ending with the tragic irony of Christopher Reeve, just months away from his real-life catastrophic spinal injury, releasing a trapped bird through an open window.

All of life so fleeting and beautiful and painful.

I cry again, so hard I can hardly see.

Where is she? *Is* she? Is there more to life than this life?

I circle back to the only thought that helps: *I can get through this if I know I will see her again.*

The idea that consciousness exists after death seems like such wishful thinking, especially when the quality of the rest of your life hinges on the truth or fallacy of the concept.

What is the truth?

There *is* an answer. That's the fact that has always plagued me. There is an answer, but so often unknowable, to every single question a person can ask.

Caitlin was 33, the Jesus age, and I am seeing 33 and 333 everywhere. On clocks when I look at them; and 33 minutes or 33 miles to every destination we plug into the GPS. Sinéad notices that Caitlin's Instagram account has 333 posts. Receipts are $33.03, $13.33. My brokenhearted post from December 21: 133 comments. Her Facebook account: 1,333 friends. Andrew's street address in Maine, 33. In a Boston café, I am reading when something makes me look up. An elegant older lady is rising from her table, wearing a sweater that is normal-looking but for the angel wings printed on the back. I open my phone to see if I can sneak a picture of them. It's 3:33.

I reason that if you begin to look for things, you will see them. You look for your husband's green cap in an airport crowd, and your eyes see all the green there is to see. I am well aware that my antennae are up, sensitive and ready to notice the slightest meaningful occurrence.

I must simply be *looking for* 333, I tell myself, when it whizzes past on a license plate.

Since childhood, I've had a singular thought in the back of my mind, and now that thought is in the forefront: *we find ourselves here.*

We humans find ourselves alive, with no explanation. Long ago, we emerged from our caves and turned so much of the natural world into everything that we now take for granted. But essentially, we are simple: we are cycle after cycle of creatures who are born, who live, and who die.

I'm pretty sure that there is no absolute proof that consciousness expires with the physical, or that brain matter creates consciousness, but I set aside the soul books and go on a search through journal articles to see what's out there.

I brace myself for proof that my doubt is well founded, but in fact I find no real insight into how or why consciousness is, only a lot of talk about how the scientific community refers to it as "the hard problem." I experience fresh appreciation for just how much people of science have figured out in a few short centuries, but I am more impressed with the universe itself, with how much humans have not come *close* to figuring out.

No, there don't seem to be definitive answers to questions of consciousness out there in the land of humans. There exist only beliefs and theories—so many of them—all populating a spectrum of evolving ideas for which there is no absolute proof.

I look up from my desk and out the window toward the maples and birches that line the river.

Trees were my first friends. It was kind of a joke in my family that Maryanne talked to trees.

We now know that the natural world is even more alive than we realized, that trees use chemical messages and electrical impulses to communicate with each other.

I wonder what I was doing when I was age three and four and talking to the trees. Are we born with some kind of sensory antennae that retract or dissolve as we age?

How much don't we know?

❦

I have never been to California, but what is probably self-preservation is pushing me to get us there, to a place bigger than our transient human selves. I think we need to see that big Pacific coast, need to stand next to redwoods older than we can ever be. Press our hands against that strong, enduring bark. Find new appreciation for living.

We book flights to Los Angeles, with plans to drive straight to Big Sur, then up the coast to San Francisco to see Jess.

At Logan Airport, I open my little travel computer for the first time since December 20 and mentally reel, seeing all the windows containing my last hopeful posts, still open. iMessages updates before my eyes, all the texts of the past few weeks flashing into view as if in real time, creating an illusion that yes, we can go back, go back and fix it, change the outcome.

As we wait for our flight to board, I receive a message from a friend of Jess's family. She has sent me a link to a medium who talks about animals and birds and signs and such. She urges me to play it, so I plug in my earphones and listen until we board. The medium says, "Ask for signs. You will get them. They will surprise you."

On the flight, I sit by the window, and as we approach the West, I look out at all the high-altitude places Caitlin, with her poor lung function, was unable to visit the past ten years—the Rocky Mountains, the Grand Canyon. I am wearing her tiny Parisian bird ring on a chain around my neck, and I squeeze the ring into my hand.

I'm so sorry life was so hard, I whisper. I look out over the clouds, as if she might appear. I don't expect anything, but I ask anyway. *How about a sign, bud?*

An hour later, we are preparing to land when a loud howling starts up in front of us. It is coming from a cat. Right there all along, in the seat directly in front of us. It seems so perfect that Nick and I look at each other and laugh.

When we stand to leave, I want to sneak a picture, but the cat is hunkered down in his carry case. I try anyway, and as I do, he sits up and looks straight at me.

Sign? I'll take it.

It is raining in California. These are hundred-year rains and they are washing out the coast north of us. They keep us in Santa Monica for a week. We are made to live inside the moments we find ourselves in. We do things we hadn't planned: see Malibu and Beverly Hills and Santa Barbara and Miles-and-Jack country.

And there is a strange, small-world, meaningful fact: our friends and neighbors from the fifteenth floor in Pittsburgh, Mary and Ralph, own a place just down the beach from our hotel. All this time, when they would go to California, I thought they were somewhere else, far away. Never having been here, I didn't have much of a map in my head.

And Mallory, the young woman with CF whom we met in Pittsburgh, who is from Beverly Hills, is in the hospital in Santa Monica. Her mother offers to meet me for coffee if I am up for it.

I am not up for much.

One evening, while Nick goes for a long walk toward the Santa Monica Pier, I watch him from our balcony, his figure growing smaller and smaller, night coming on. At the pier, the Ferris wheel lights up and spins vibrant flashing neon out into the dark. In another life, we would be there as a family, riding the coaster, playing arcade games. Caitlin at seven, at ten, at fifteen, all those ages now one holographic, multidimensional image.

I throw myself onto the bed and cry and cry.

I will never be able to stop crying.

I am getting a pedicure in my Santa Monica hotel and it is the slowest one in the world. I try to relax as the technician works on my left foot, but all I can think of is how horrifying and ultimately needless had been that partial amputation. I keep picturing Caitlin and me getting pedicures together at various points in our life—in Boston or on vacations in Miami, and later, when I pushed her in the wheelchair over to the Pittsburgh Fairmont's spa for a little pampering.

Her last pedicures I did myself, on her bed, because she no longer had the energy to go to a salon. The past year, I gave her leg and foot massages almost every day because it was the only thing that gave her relief from the nearly constant painful body aching the oxygen–carbon dioxide imbalance caused her.

I don't want to start crying in front of the pedicurist, so I half-heartedly look through the basket of predictable women's magazines. But—a surprise. Tucked in there is a *New York Times Magazine* from the end of November, with a cover story on Martin Scorsese titled "On Faith." I'd brought that particular one into the hospital to give to Caitlin, because she had a deep appreciation of his movies. I'd never gotten around to reading it. I wonder now if she had.

The article is about Scorsese's new film, *Silence*, and about his life-long contemplation of the nature of faith. I wonder what Caitlin would have thought of the film. It had received mixed reviews, but Caitlin's opinion would have been the opinion I would have been interested in. She had a keen ability to analyze and to consider, with empathy, the most complicated subjects. See things other people didn't see.

I thought of her fascination with Tolstoy's *A Confession*, and Tolstoy's ultimate acceptance of the paradox of faith.

I'm not quite there yet. I'm not anywhere.

After the pedicure, I walk out onto the beach. Down near the water is a big flock of seagulls. I walk past them, telling myself I can't desperately look at every bird in the world, hoping for a sign.

But I see that the one closest to me is standing on one leg. He stands on it for so long that I think perhaps he has only one leg.

None of the other gulls is standing like that. I keep watching and waiting for him to move and find myself getting all choked up and happy and talking to Caitlin. *Is that you, buddy? Is that you?*

She feels real and close for those moments and I think, *This is what you're going to have to do: take whatever portal is open, whenever you can.*

Big Sur helps us, with its wild, winding coast road that splits the jagged cliffs from the vast Pacific. Its forests are deep and hushed, filled with shade and dappled light and birdsong, and there are heady scents of earth and tree resins and ocean air. Big Sur is a sanctuary, it is nature's cathedral. We walk along pine-needle paths, and Nick carries a photo of Caitlin that he positions in tree boughs and on rocks. He carries a cloth drawstring bag that contains the religious artifacts people sent to the ICU: the crucifix, the Star of David, the Celtic cross, and positions them around her photograph to create small, pleasing tableaus that manage to connect her to this trip in a way that feels physical.

So the glorious days here are somewhat easy. But night is still night, and nights are hard. At 2:00 a.m., after falling asleep to a dozen messages from people—many of them strangers—telling me of signs they are sure they received from Caitlin's soul (!) (How can they be so sure?), I come awake.

I slip out of bed, wondering if Jess was awake ten hours ago, when it was 2:00 a.m. in Kenya. We have taken to calling this sleepless time of night the witching hour. She and Andrew have gone over to Kenya to work at the girls' school for the couple of months that Jess can be away from her own medical team. She will be returning soon and we plan on seeing her in San Francisco.

The fireplace glows red with the last embers of our fire, lighting my way as I step out onto our balcony and into a bowl of stars. For a moment, the exhilaration I've always felt at the sight of a bright night sky fills me. Then I step a little farther and it is as if I fall out of my body. I see my own brief spark of existence. Dust to dust. Over forever.

Back in bed, I lie with tears sliding down my face and into my mouth. I wedge a pillow next to my head to create a wall so that the glow from my cell phone won't wake Nick. I check my email and see that Andrew has forwarded me a couple of emails he had received from Caitlin not long ago. I read the first one.

With my big book, *Sarum*—that I've been reading that traces England from beginning of man to now—to this new book I'm reading—which does a similar thing with the slave trade and is already so good and opening up new ways of looking at slavery (for me) I just feel like alongside this election, which is challenging everything I took for granted . . . it's an interesting and weird time to be alive and experiencing. I can't help but imagine these times in the past that I read about, and then think how the time we live in now will just be something that happened to someone else, in the future. . . . It will be this weird blip in history that is a foregone conclusion because it's over, it's sorted out. We learn about bad things that happened and somehow they don't seem quite as unbelievable because the people in the future have figured out why it happens, and we know the ending. I hope it doesn't happen soon, but at some point the US will no longer be around, or it will be much different than it is now. And it won't seem weird to people reading about it in history books. We will just seem like the dumb idiots of history who messed things up. A question on a test somewhere. We parse the decades out and they all seem so different.

When I read *Sarum*, I have a tendency to do a double take when things are different—from, say 1650 to 1690—when the area in the book has undergone a huge change. But of course in our modern history entire revolutions and wars happen in shorter times. Countries fall. We are all the same and we all have a collective fallibility and vulnerability. It can happen to any country and any place . . . but we also are all the same in that we never seem to really learn from history or believe we are the ones making mistakes.

It's part of why the idea of souls makes sense to me. This place is just like a ropes course for souls. A learning center. It never changes and the collective body of humans can never sustain their progress too too much or else there is not enough to challenge the souls. *Imagine all the people living life in peace—John Lennon* 🐇—well that wouldn't really work if you believe we need to be challenged to grow. At least in the human form.

A ropes course for souls. How perfectly put. And a comfort, coming directly from Caitlin, when I need it most.

I think of how easily she and I had accepted the theory of re-incarnation. We even had a joke—if we came across a person who was rigid, shallow, insufferable, we might give him or her a bit of a pass. *Oh, he's just a young soul, he can't help it.* "Young soul" became a shortcut phrase we could use to quickly describe someone in a way that said it all, yet in a tolerant, compassionate way.

Reincarnation had made sense to me, but now I'm desperate and don't trust my judgment. I'm a grieving mother whose daughter's existence is on the line.

I think, okay, I'm going to ask for a hard sign. Something very specific, like the mediums suggest. I say it aloud. "I want a monarch butterfly to fly around me in a complete circle. Tomorrow."

From: Caitlin
To: Andrew
Date: July 25, 2016
Subject: Zoomed out

This article sums up everything I think about the state of the world and life and how I think—only this guy articulately wrote it and has all the facts at his fingertips to back it up. I am only an amateur historian. With all I know cobbled together from years of art history combined with an obsession with organizing time in my head—decades, centuries, eras. The entire thing has always been a visual structure in my head. Some day I will draw it for you. When I picture us now in 2016, I pull back. I always pull back and picture myself in time and in space geographically. It makes me removed enough (like this guy) to ultimately feel that there is not much I can do to change the shifts of the world, but also inspired enough to think—what is my role in this lifetime (whether it's my only lifetime or one of many, doesn't matter) to survive this time?

I am fascinated by this kind of thing. By the ebbs and flows of history. By patterns and by people and all of the stuff he talks about. I guess it's harder for many people to think in that zoomed out way. For me—it was a mechanism I cultivated as a way to deal with being sick . . . I'd zoom out, see my own smallness, realize it's all been done before and will be done again, and I could relax, and enjoy my life now. Like why I like graveyards. And reading about the Holocaust. I like reading and thinking about the ebbs and flows of human suffering, living, dying, living again. . . .

I don't think it matters if this guy is "right" about Brexit or whatever the defining moment will prove to be . . . or even if this time really will end up being a catastrophic time (ahead of us). I kind of feel it might be. But I think his way of thinking is a good one that I relate to a lot. And wish more people did. But then, we wouldn't have the same world.

. . . .

✦

In the morning, Nick and I drive down the coast road to the Esalen retreat for massages and to experience their famous hot sulfur springs. Esalen has been around since 1962, and *Mad Men*, a show Caitlin and I admired tremendously, used a fictionalized Esalen for its series finale.

Sitting in the sulfur water with the sea crashing below us, all I can think is, *It's Sunday. Exactly four weeks ago today, Caitlin was in surgery and we were so relieved and happy. And now I am at Esalen, a place that seemed like Neverland.*

Nick loves the energy at Esalen and, after his massage, walks across the property to check out the big farm garden they cultivate. I sit in an Adirondack chair overlooking the Pacific and think about Don Draper coming to know his purpose at the end of *Mad Men*, and how I wish Caitlin could see that I am there, and a couple of monarch butterflies begin flying all around . . . not tight around my face, the way I'd envisioned, but in big swooping circles that take in much more than me.

✦

San Francisco is cold with driving rain, and Kenley happens to be there for work and we take her and Jess out to dinner in the Marina district, where Jess lives. It is good to be with two of Caitlin's oldest and closest friends but we are all disembodied, only partly there, because how is it that the four of us are in San Francisco eating maccaronara and little gem salads without Caitlin when we were in Pittsburgh just minutes ago, where waiting for transplant had become the only reality?

At our hotel, there is an oval meditation pool with ninety-five-degree water and ancient Chinese *erhu* melodies playing out of speakers hidden inside shrubbery. There are tree boughs overhead that cradle the pool, and one night it rains and the rain is so beautiful it mixes with our crying and becomes the same thing.

In the daylight we drive north with Jess, dodging two hawks that fly at our windows, up to Point Reyes, where we sit at a picnic table, bundled up against the freezing cold, and eat delicious barbecued oysters and hot buttered bread. We talk about how Caitlin wrote about goodness and believed in it, deeply, without sentimentality or piety.

It seems incredibly important to create something meaningful in her honor. An idea has come to me: a portable healing garden. What is a portable healing garden? I am not yet sure.

·······

We are home from California and I look up Elisabeth Kübler-Ross's five stages of grief to see if I agree with them.

They are denial, anger, bargaining, depression, and acceptance.

Denial, yes. Denial is constant. Anger? No, not really. Where are the missing stages? Infinite sadness, where's that? And where is fear and where is anxiety and where is regret and guilt? Where is recognition of the grief loop?

I've experienced death in my life, but this is Caitlin, my sidekick, my *person*. This is my mostly companion. The one I always knew I could not live without.

With each bout of hysterical crying, you eventually cry yourself out and lie still. You become hyperconscious of your physical body.

The heart beats. The breath moves in and out.

You wonder how many breaths are left. How many heartbeats.

I do not want to live in a world where Caitlin recedes into the past, a world where she died twenty years ago.

Yet I do not want to want to die.

I ask the universe for my hour of unconsciousness and fall asleep.

Nick has gone to his office, and I realize that this is the first day I will spend alone in our house since we left Pittsburgh. I manage to take a shower, but mainly I cry all morning. My eyes sting from the daily crying, but I can't stop. Who knew a human could cry so much?

I finally decide to watch a movie that I love, *Hereafter*.

Hereafter came out in 2010 but didn't do well, mainly, I think, because people went to it expecting a disaster movie—it opens with incredible special effects that depict the 2004 Indian Ocean tsunami.

But it's not about special effects. It's an intelligent, engrossing, and well-written movie that ruminates on whether there is an afterlife. There are three interconnected stories, and Matt Damon plays the part of a reluctant medium very well.

At the end, I watch the credits and realize that it was written by Peter Morgan, writer of *The Queen* and *The Crown*. No wonder it's so good.

The last show Caitlin and I ever watched in Pittsburgh was

The Crown. We finished it right before she went into the hospital that November. At the time, I looked up some of the actual events that took place in the show, including the queen's friendship with "Porchie," and came upon this statement she made after his death: *Nothing that can be said can begin to take away the anguish and the pain of these moments*, she wrote. *Grief is the price we pay for love*.

She was, in turn, quoting from Dr. Colin Murray Parkes, the hospice pioneer who wrote, *The pain of grief is just as much part of life as the joy of love: it is perhaps the price we pay for love, the cost of commitment. To ignore this fact, or to pretend that it is not so, is to put on emotional blinkers which leave us unprepared for the losses that will inevitably occur in our own lives and unprepared to help others cope with losses in theirs.*

<hr />

We are so exposed after our deaths, especially when death is un-expected, all of our bits and pieces left behind for others to see. Caitlin once told me I could write what I needed to, if I ever needed to, but I set myself the limits I think she would have agreed with. I have access to her email but won't read any correspondence that others don't share with me first.

Finances are another story. I open her computer to try and make sense of her accounts and see that she kept little windows open on her computer, where she would jot down thoughts, lists, reminders.

I'll be right back, those windows promise.

I open the drawer in her desk in Boston. It's messy with pens and notecards and hair bands and stamps and old mail, and stuffed into the back corner is a folded piece of paper. On the outside she had written, *Fear Exercise*.

Fear Exercise confesses her terror of me dying, a phobia she'd had since seeing the Roald Dahl movie *The Witches*, when she was seven years old. Before that movie, she had never been bothered by daycare, or by us leaving her with sitters.

The scene that traumatized her is dramatic, with barely any dialogue. In it, we see the parents of young Luke getting ready to go out for the night. His mother puts on her scarf, says good-bye to him and his grandmother, and leaves with his father. In the morning Luke knocks on their bedroom door. The bed has not been slept in. He wanders the house calling for them as a police car pulls up outside. A police officer approaches the door, holding the folded scarf. He knocks.

Forever after that film, Caitlin was terrified of losing us—of losing me, specifically. As tough as she was, as self-sufficient, she needed me, needed *someone* who would put everything aside to help her. Facing critical illness can be terrifying. To face it without help would be exponentially worse.

※

You don't know me, but . . .
You haven't met me, but . . .
I hope you don't mind, but . . .

The messages come and come. Emails, blog comments, private messages, USPS buckets stuffed with cards and letters and gifts of cat and bird ornaments and books of poetry and art and daily affirmations. One package contains a bag of beautiful metal charms engraved with Caitlin's bird-on-a-branch drawing, which I'd used for the cover of the service program and published on the blog.

Astonishing! Such kindness. Such connection. I savor every message, the words that keep her alive for a little while longer for the moments it takes to read them. They inspire me to keep writing about her—why not, if it helps people so much? It's the one thing I can do that feels right.

I have never met you or Caitlin, but reading about her positive outlooks on life gives me strength. I struggle with my own issues every day, but sometimes I read her writings that you post for a little bit of guidance. I just wanted to tell you this so you know that she continues to touch more lives than you may know.

Thank you for sharing your stories of Caitlin's amazing life. I think of when you told us she tipped generously so that's what I have been doing whenever I go out to eat. It is fun and I think of Caitlin when I do.

I've written before about connections—between people, animals, nature, events. It can't be scientifically explained, but they are everywhere, and I feel the most peace when I wonder about them. Your writing through this blog has allowed me to feel so many connections with people I've never known. It's like what a great novel does: we get to know and love the characters like they were in our own lives, like we have had experiences and memories with them. You've allowed that with Caitlin and all the other "characters" in your "story." Yet, all of these people are real, and so our connection to them is real, strengthened by your honest writing, the pictures and videos, the text messages, the program from her service. So, is literature allowing us to mimic these connections that we should have in our real lives? So much about your writing has made me ask big questions.

Hundreds of people are reaching out and there is a massive contingency of your daughter's amazing friends that have been texting about her and thinking about her impressive life. It's a small world and so many connections your daughter had and continue to flourish because of her. Know that people love the updates because it made them feel a part of her fight just like Caitlin was a part of our lives as we went through growing up.

I cannot tell you enough how much I, and I'm sure many others, value your open honesty. I am still in therapy and we often talk about the loss I suffered at age twenty. So much of what you describe, I remember keenly, but was not really old enough to process or metabolize properly.

I hid it all.

To get to Boston from our house, you take the Mass Turnpike east. The turnpike passes under an overpass labeled Grove Street. If you look to the right and through the trees you will see Edgell Grove Cemetery.

We will always see Edgell Grove Cemetery on our way to Boston.

I am driving there and I've decided to take the advice of people and talk aloud to Caitlin. As I drive past the overpass, I say, "So I'm trying to talk to you, buddy. And I'm wondering what it's like where you are and what you're doing. And I'm wondering if it's true that animals have souls, then is Hobo there? My dog from when I was little?"

And not one minute later, a box truck passes me on the left, four giant letters painted on its side: HOBO.

Is a coincidence what the dictionary tells me it is?—"a remarkable concurrence of events or circumstances without apparent causal connection." Or are we talking about Carl Jung's synchronicities, occurrences that do not appear to be causally related but to which there seem to be meaningful connections? Is "seem" the operative word? Does the universe operate on a principle of synchronicity?

I know one thing: you can't make this stuff up.

One of Caitlin's Friends of Prouty Garden collaborators, Shelley, checks in with me. *Hi Maryanne, How are you? That was what Caitlin usually texted me with and it was something of a revelation to me—three small words that said so much. "I'm thinking of you, I care about you, I want to hear about your life, I want to be in touch with you." I started texting my friends more often just with, "How are you?" and our relationships felt immediately so much closer.*

During our back-and-forth she says, *I have to tell you I am seeing a medium on Wednesday. I've never been, but one sort of popped up on Yelp after Caitlin died and I felt compelled to make an appointment.*

A medium? I'm not sure I like this idea. I don't want to hear that Caitlin didn't "show." I don't want to know that there's nothing. Shelley didn't even know Caitlin all that well.

Shelley tells me the medium's name, Sirrý, and says that she is very well regarded. I look up Sirrý's website. It is full of information and frequently asked questions. There's a whole page on how to protect yourself from frauds. Sirrý points out that she hopes one session will be enough for a grieving person, that she believes it best not to become dependent on mediums. She's also, apparently, been vetted by an organization called Forever Family Foundation, which has rigorously blind-tested mediums. From the Forever Family site: *The mediums listed on this page have had their abilities evaluated under controlled conditions. These mediums are listed purely as a resource for*

the bereaved, and certification is based only on a medium's proficiency.
Mediums listed have not paid to appear on this site, and the certification
evaluation is conducted free of charge.

I count only twenty-seven mediums they've deemed worthy of
certification in all of the United States.

⁂

February 1, 2017

SHELLEY: Maryanne, Caitlin came through loud and clear the
whole time and had so much to say. I will be getting the recording
within the next day or so and will give you much more info. I was
just sort of experiencing it and it's all just this incredible blur. But
she said you took amazing care of her and she knows how deeply
you are grieving, like your chest has been ripped open.
Sirrý is Icelandic! She has lived all over the world. She is not
always familiar with American customs or geography. But she
was really wonderful and gifted. It was amazing to watch her
work, like she was listening to someone, and then she'd say,
"okay, okay, got it," and then try to describe to me what she
was getting—but it's almost like detective work, trying to figure
out what exactly she was being shown or told and what the
significance was.

What I feel: relief. For all the obvious reasons.
Then, curiosity. A little glimmer of hope.
Shelley signs off by offering to send me the recording when she
receives it from Sirrý.
Two hours later, my friend Susan arrives for a visit. It is late

afternoon, about 4:00 p.m. I open the door to join her outside and to let Henry out.

We hear and feel the beating of large wings behind us and duck instinctively, then Susan clutches my arm as a red-tailed hawk glides over our heads. It flies low over the garden and disappears beyond the far wall.

Our eyes lock. *What just happened?*

It was as if it had been sitting on the roof of the house, waiting.

"I'm so glad I was here because it's the kind of thing you would try to tell someone and it would be hard to believe," Susan says.

Later, she texts me: *It really did feel like that hawk wanted our attention. It really did. Never in my life have I had a hawk come that close to me.*

I hadn't yet told people about my hawk experiences. I planned to hold on to those stories and write some kind of hawk post at some point.

I never did. I saved the hawks for now.

Shelley sends her recording and I listen, afraid at first, then transfixed. Sirrý gets the name right, asks, "Do you understand a name like Cayla, Caitlin?" And does Shelley understand that "this life was cut short, a quick, sudden passing, unexpected"?

Sirrý says, "It feels to me that either I am crushed from the side, or there's an impact on my side . . . do you understand that there would have been an impact in some way that her head would have been impacted? She's pushing on my head, I'm having this massive headache in my head. If that makes sense? Massive impact or massive pressure on my head."

I'm listening to this and remembering Caitlin's words, *I've always thought I was going to die of a stroke.*

Sirrý asks if Caitlin collapsed, as there were people working on her chest.

Shelley says that Caitlin had been waiting for a lung transplant.

"But the final thing was the pressure on her head?"

Shelley confirms this. "Yes. A brain bleed."

I am so terrified of having a stroke like that. Locked-in syndrome. I am so so afraid of it in ways I can't even be ok with.

Sirrý talks dates, about how Caitlin got really sick in November, but had been sick for two years. Then the talk gets a little trippy because apparently Caitlin is listening to David Bowie: "I'm listening to him in the universe. Damn good concert."

Damn good concert. That's a Caitlin phrase.

Sirrý asks, "Would it make sense to hear, 'Two days before my passing I got the green light'? She shows me, 'Here we are, and 2 days before I die, I got the green light. We thought all was good.'"

Got the green light. Again, Caitlin's way of speaking.

Sirrý then says that Caitlin wants Shelley to teach her daughter a David Bowie song, and begins humming "Across the Universe." She corrects herself, confused, and says, "No, that's not a David Bowie song."

Shelley says, "That's a Beatles song."

Sirrý asks more questions Shelley can't answer. Did Caitlin's parents cut a piece of her hair? There's to be a Jim Morrison type of shrine where she will be laid to rest? Lots of stones?

Shelley tells her that she's pretty sure we are planning to build a private mausoleum.

Sirrý says that in her fifteen or sixteen years of doing this work, she's never been shown a mausoleum.

Shelley felt a strong bond with Caitlin but she didn't know Caitlin all that well. Their total time together, in person, added up to a couple of hours. She didn't know details. So a lot of what Sirrý had said, Shelley could not confirm. Which also meant that any online search of Shelley would never reveal the details that Sirrý provided.

Later, I tell Shelley that David Bowie did record the Beatles' "Across the Universe." That the nurse did cut pieces of Caitlin's hair after she died. That we had visited Père Lachaise Cemetery in Paris in 2004, and had seen Jim Morrison's notorious grave, and that Père Lachaise had inspired Caitlin to want a mausoleum.

Perhaps Sirrý has a way of tapping in, energetically, to what has existed, and what has happened. Or perhaps her ability is what it seems to be and the essence of Caitlin, her consciousness, her *soul*, really does endure.

How are you?

We get the question all the time. There are so many ways to answer: okay, horrible, up and down. Hoping in the veracity of souls, then despairing at the idea.

We decide on the word "functioning." We're functioning, we say.

I picture "functioning" as a sine wave. The sine wave moves up and down and forward and that's how we live: functioning, existing, okay one hour, not so good the next, but flowing forward, forward flowing.

Functioning means we are showering and keeping our house clean and eating and working, sort of, and crying, and lying prone, staring at the ceiling.

Functioning means we are human contradictions: even when we are smiling and having a good time, we're not.

※

I begin to see hawks constantly, and in strange places. Over Whole Foods. Flying low across Route 9, right in front of my windshield. Sitting in our trees. Landing on the median strip of a busy highway.

Hawks are apparently a "thing" after death. Messengers. A friend tells me that for a week after her niece died horribly and tragically, a hawk sat on a fence post in the family's backyard. Same spot, every day. Just sat there.

One afternoon, I have been having an extra hard day. I am on my bed crying, head swimming with doubt and missing and pain. I think about the fact that my brain might be unconsciously searching the sky for hawks. And it might unconsciously be looking at clocks at precisely thirty-three minutes past each hour, the way you can wake yourself up without an alarm.

I sit up on my bed and say aloud, "You can't expect to see hawks flying all around you all the time just because you're in need of one!"

An instant later there's a white flash, a commotion outside our second-story bedroom. I run to the window. Two hawks are out there, flying low and crazy-close to the house.

I've lived at this property since I was twenty-six years old. I've never seen this kind of hawk behavior. I stand at the window and watch them, wondering if this can possibly be just a coincidence.

I'm aware of my vulnerability, my desire to believe, so it seems best to remain indecisive, to stand apart and wait for unquestionable proof. To fall back onto the bed and give in to misery.

※

I call them my List of the Familiars, actions that were so much the fabric of my days that the realization that I will never do them again is part of the shock after shock of all this. Snap the sterile caps off the vials of ceftazidime and sterile water. Clean the tops with alcohol wipes. Unwrap a syringe. Draw it back to prep it. Insert the needle into the water vial, draw it back to remove all 10ccs. Push the water into the ceftazidime vial. Shake. Draw 5ccs of medicine up then push it into a clean nebulizer cup. Screw the cover onto the cup, insert the filter lid, add the mouthpiece. Set it on the living room side table, by her nebulizer for her morning dose. Cover the vial and refrigerate for the evening dose. Rinse berries, chop kale and red cabbage and papaya, mix it all in the blender with almond milk ice cream and coconut water. Pour it into a glass, cap it and refrigerate for her breakfast. Wash the blender. Count out seven digestive enzymes. Take an inventory of meds while I'm at it. Take last evening's used neb cups apart, rinse them, put them in a bowl to await sterilization. Every two days, boil a big pot of water. Drop the four nebulizer cup parts in and set the timer for ten minutes. Drain the water. Lay out clean paper towel. Shake each part to help it dry. Carefully and lightly wrap the four parts of each cup into a clean paper towel. Store the clean cups in a bowl. Lift an empty oxygen tank onto the tank filler. Click it into place and turn it on. After it fills, open the valve to ensure that it's really full. Fill all the empty tanks. Drive to Whole Foods to get there when it opens at 8am. The parking lot will have spaces and Caitlin will be safely asleep, Mary and Ralph right next door in case of an emergency if Nick or Andrew are not in town. Gather up the staples she will go through in days: sweet potatoes, broccoli, greens, papayas, berries, eggs, coconut water, almond milk ice cream, frozen berries, almond milk pudding, cheese sticks, beet ravioli, more B2, protein powder, a nagging thought, Is she out of magnesium? Better get some. Swing by CVS for two giant big bags of whatever meds she's out of this week. Prep her lunch and snacks and dinner. Do chest PT. Do it again where she feels herself to be clogged.

Prepare for an outing: set up the wheelchair, the tanks, a juice box and protein bar in case of blood sugar dives. Don't dare get in the elevator without two extra oxygen tanks. Check that those tanks are really full. Double check. Push her into the elevator and down to the car, help her and her tank into the passenger seat, fold up the wheelchair, lift it into the rear of the car. Arrive, pull out the chair, snap it open, set down the chair cushion, loop the extra oxygen tank carrier straps over the handles. Wheel it to the passenger door. Lift out the oxygen tank, hold it steady while she settles in. Prop the tank on the footrest. Kiss the top of her head.

⁂

You want to do nothing. You want to roll over and go back to sleep, want to exist with no expectations or responsibilities.

You can't. Living means doing.

Nick and I were careful to set up our own wills in case Caitlin was ever left on her own, but she had no will so we must sit through the grim business of working with our lawyer to fill out the paperwork and file probate to gain control of her small estate.

Ironically—because everything is now ironic—our lawyer's office is in the same building that houses the Massachusetts office of the Cystic Fibrosis Foundation.

We work with Rick and I see just how muddled my head is. It's not just the legalities. My head is muddled from not having lived in our house for a few years, and from knowing that the Pittsburgh apartment is still full of our two years' worth of *stuff*, and that Caitlin's Boston apartment is waiting for our attention, too.

My sister and her husband offer to go to Pittsburgh and pack it up, but Nick and I are in agreement. Packing up feels like something we need to do. We decide that all four of us will go and that we will take Henry. He seems a necessary part of the process. Then

Nick and I will continue on to another escape, the Arizona desert, where we can hike and see stars.

I am packing for the trip when an email from L.L.Bean informs me that those back-ordered scuffs, the red ones with the cat silhouette, which I'd ordered for Caitlin and forgotten, have been shipped to Pittsburgh.

An hour later, I am rinsing dishes and realize that the candle from Caitlin's last birthday cake at home is tucked into a little vase on the windowsill.

Life is a minefield.

⁂

The Pittsburgh apartment is a time capsule, the rooms neat and orderly, just as we left them. It is all so dear and familiar, as if we could slide right back into our everyday rhythms.

At one point I am alone there. I walk into the kitchen and call into Caitlin's bedroom, "Can I get you anything, bud? Are you ready for your shake?"

My voice breaks and I slide to the floor, thinking about how I could simply stay down there and refuse to recover. I could keep pretending she is on the other side of that wall.

Henry trots over, curious. Sniffing, hoping for food. I burst into tears and hug him. Then I get myself up off the floor and try to sort through drawers. But I can't focus. And when my eyes find Nick's, his are drifting about as vacantly as mine. He is as hopeless as I am.

My sister and her husband take over. They are natural workers and are soon breaking everything down, packing boxes, labeling them, the apartment looking less and less like ours until . . . it no longer is.

While we are in Pittsburgh, Katie has an appointment in New Hampshire. Pregnant with her second child and sick with grief, Katie had contemplated seeing a medium named Karissa, whose name and good reputation she kept coming across. She decided to see a psychologist instead, but the psychologist surprised her by suggesting a visit with a medium. The psychologist wrote down a contact and slipped the paper across her desk and there was Karissa's name. That decided it.

I am doubly interested because Katie is the most unsearchable person I know. She dislikes social media, spent much of the previous decade living abroad, and has zero internet presence. I search her name locked inside parentheses to see what comes up and find just a brief mention in a directory for a job she once had at a university.

We are still in Pittsburgh the day of Kate's appointment. That night she emails me and attaches her typed-up transcript. She writes that she heard from her father's father and brother, her Spanish husband's grandmother, *some woman who I can't figure out who she is*, and her grammy Mary. She says the section relating to her father was particularly uncanny, that the reading went very well, but when she had been more than halfway into her hour-long session she'd been feeling disappointed that Caitlin hadn't come through. Karissa said she could ask the others to gently step back and let the desired person in. When she did so, Caitlin apparently had appeared, looking as if she were in her early twenties.

I am a bit suspect to hear that Katie had to ask for Caitlin but the rest of the transcribed conversation is information that couldn't come from guessing, starting with Karissa telling Katie that there was a real sense of helplessness surrounding Caitlin's passing. "It's not like there wasn't treatment but there wasn't enough treatment.

She's showing me that treatment has only progressed so far to treat specifically what she had. Something very progressive in her body, cancer-like but not that, more rare."

Katie said yes, she understood that, then told Karissa it was interesting that Karissa found Caitlin looking as she had in her twenties. She'd had several dreams about Caitlin, and in all of them she looked as she had in her twenties.

Karissa said this was common, that people present themselves as they were when they looked and felt their best. As she spoke, "Caitlin" was apparently agreeing, and saying she could run again. Then she made a joke about her hair, saying it was long and pretty again, and that fact startled Katie so much that she interrupted.

"Her *hair*?"

Caitlin's hair vanity had been a lifelong source of humor among the three of us.

Karissa said, "Like is there a joke about someone not being able to braid hair? Or some sort of a joke here? It feels like toward the end, it feels like she was someone who was naturally very pretty and she's showing me that toward the end that shifted for her, and I'm getting the sense of her saying, 'Fix my hair, okay, somebody come and fix my hair!'"

This was true, and a weird thing to simply invent, and it sounded exactly like Caitlin.

I let myself process that.

As the reading progressed, Karissa said she didn't know why but Caitlin kept pointing out the number four as significant.

Katie said she didn't know what that meant either, and Karissa replied, "I have to just give you the four and hope that it makes sense later."

Karissa then said, "So she wants me to call you her sister. She's saying, 'This is my sister, this is my sister.'" And that Caitlin wanted to talk about a little boy, whom Karissa assumed was Katie's little boy. Caitlin was saying she was "still an aunt, still involved," and that she was able to influence him to be mischievous.

"And she keeps wanting to come back to her illness and tell me it's genetic," Karissa said. "Did you know that?" Kate said yes, yes, and Karissa said, "This is why she's at peace."

Karissa also brings up me, and my close relationship with Caitlin, and that Caitlin feels present in our lives and can hear our thoughts, that she still feels like she's a part of everything and hasn't missed a thing.

The transcript ends with Karissa saying, "Okay, she's laughing at your husband. Hold on here. Does he speak another language?"

Katie explained that her husband grew up in Spain, and Karissa said, "Okay, she's laughing at him trying to get certain words right. 'They are literally like Lucy and Ricky.'"

Lucy and Ricky Ricardo, our lifelong tap tap buddies. And the psychic's "four," the transplant that finally happened on the fourth offer.

It's comforting, as the other medium was comforting, but it's all still hard to fully believe. Why? Because it seems so magical, so fantastical? As I start to close the email, I see that Kate added a PS to the bottom of the transcript.

So here my recording cut off! But we were almost done anyway. Karissa told me that she was getting the symbol of an open book, and that's the sign that the spirit is open to questions, so I asked if Caitlin had met the new baby—she laughed and said "oh yes" right away. In fact, she has been playing with her! Caitlin said the new baby hasn't fully "dropped in" and is back and forth and that she is holding and playing with her.

Karissa also mentioned that three giant angelic beings were

waiting next to Caitlin as she stood beside her hospital bed and that they ushered her passing. She said that there was suffering, but that she herself didn't suffer. Karissa saw a coma-like state and said that Caitlin had already "detached" by the time it was time for her to pass. She was ready to pass.

·❦·

In a dovetail coincidence, it turned out that Mallory, the young woman from California, had been officially listed for transplant at UPMC the day we arrived in Pittsburgh.

She and her mother are staying in the Fairmont Hotel two blocks away while they wait to move into an apartment. I don't plan to see them—I shrink from it, imagining that it would be disturbing for them to see us and think about what can go wrong when they are newly so desperate for transplant to go right. But Nick thinks it will be good for them to know people in this city, so he invites them to the gathering of friends and neighbors that Mary and Ralph have planned for us for Sunday, our final day.

The gathering is in Ralph and Mary's apartment, across the hall from ours. I wait until it's under way before I go over. Henry trots over beside me, at home in Pittsburgh as if nothing has changed, but I feel as if I'm stepping sideways, as if I'm already gone.

Mallory arrives after me, wheeling her oxygen tank behind her tall, lanky frame. She has grown thinner since October. I can feel the bones of her rib cage when I hug her. I am nervous for her and the cepacia fevers that plague her, but I assure her that she won't have to wait as long as Caitlin. I tell her that her height is a gift.

She is cautious, hopeful. The past few months have been hard on her. She is only twenty-four but exudes the wisdom and compassion of someone far older. She is empathic and bright, a straight-A

Stanford grad, avid surfer, passionate writer. I want her to have a long life and I look around at all the good Pittsburgh people who were here for us, and who will be, I know, here for the Smiths. It's going to go well for you, I say. "What happened to Caitlin came from the wait. You can be very hopeful."

Not that long ago, when there was no transplant option, people with end-stage cystic fibrosis waited only to die. At least our waiting let us live with hope.

❦

Our departure from Pittsburgh has a soundtrack. I wake up and realize it's the twentieth—two months, how can it be? Our packed bags wait by the door. We shower, dress, and as Nick calls the elevator, I take one last look before I close the door on our Pittsburgh life.

It's 6:00 a.m., still dark, still quiet. Our driver, a man Nick trusted and used the past two years, is downstairs waiting, and we climb into his back seat. As we merge onto the 376 on-ramp, Jim tells us that although it is difficult for him to talk about hard things, he needs us to know that we inspired him, that witnessing the support of all our friends and family during our time in Pittsburgh made a strong impression on him.

"Your daughter was teaching herself guitar," he says. A statement. "Yes," I say.

He tells us that after picking us up at the airport earlier in the week, he was inspired to do something he'd long planned to do, ever since he lost his own brother to cancer. The two used to play guitar together, and for twenty years, Jim had been meaning to record their favorite song.

He had finally done it. "I'd like to play it for you," he says, "and if you like it, I'll send it to you."

Nick and I clutch hands as Jim's recording of "The Sound of Silence" fills the car. An acoustic arrangement that is perfect, beautiful. I feel disconnected, as if I am inside a film, watching us. Nick passes me a tissue, and as we speed along the dark highway, high in the sky is a waning crescent moon, inverse to the waxing crescent moon that hung outside the medical jet when we flew to Pittsburgh, three years earlier, so full of hope for a swift and successful transplant.

Our flight to Phoenix departs from gate thirty-three.

❦

We are migrants in the land of grief. After desert hiking in Arizona, we find ourselves beachside in Florida, at a hotel with an atmosphere that feels like our beloved Virgin Islands. Soft reggae plays in the background. There are palm trees and thatched buildings and the water is a Caribbean turquoise.

Nick has gone for a walk and I am sitting by the pool when I happen to check Facebook. From a post, I see that Heather is so recovered from her transplant that she, too, is in Florida. She is at Disney World.

I've never been one to say that life's not fair, or to be angry about Caitlin's CF, or her not-inevitable rapid decline and need for a lung transplant. I've always tried to be philosophical and optimistic, and I truly do believe that tough experiences make you a more compassionate human being.

But.

I drink a rum punch for lunch. And then I drink another one.

And I watch people. Families with adult children. Mothers and daughters. I imagine her here—ambling in her slow way across the pool deck. I see her big sunglasses, her long hair, and I keep thinking I was a fool to have had 100 percent faith that the transplant would happen and that she would prevail.

I want to go back and cherish every minute even more than I did. I post a photograph and tell people, *Run and hug the people you love. Right now.*

Nick begins to plan the private mausoleum. He's secured an oak-covered knoll that faces west in the garden cemetery. We send out a call for heart-shaped rocks to use in the mausoleum's construction. They begin to arrive from everywhere.

Those who examine the cognitive science behind bereavement say that "sensed presences" are normal parts of grief. British researchers Edith Steffen and Adrian Coyle wrote that linking bereavement research with research into posttraumatic cognitive processes has drawn attention to the significance of postbereavement "meaning-making." It's what we humans do.

And most of us have experienced the "frequency illusion," whereby you hear about a thing and then see it referenced immediately afterward.

But those explanations don't demystify the synchronicities that fly at me like fireflies on a summer's night, so I book an appointment with Karissa, the New Hampshire medium Katie saw.

I meet her on a bright April afternoon. She is younger than I imagined—thirty or so—with large, clear, intelligent eyes and a warm, bubbly manner. She is an easy person to meet, but I am nervous. I feel like this session will be decisive. Caitlin is either out there or she's not and maybe I am about to know for sure. But Kate's experience was uncanny, and I'm very curious about the postscript part—that Caitlin's soul had detached before passing. The truth is, I'm haunted by the suffering we witnessed, and it would be comforting to believe she hadn't been truly present. A detached soul at the end sounds like that certainty I'd had as a child, that I'd be able to "jump out of my body" if the physical became too much to bear.

I take a seat in Karissa's sunny office, and she explains how she works. She says that she doesn't control who comes through, that sometimes it can be someone from your past whom you barely remember, but she wants me to know that whoever comes through is never a mistake.

I knew this already, from Kate's experience. "Okay," I say, determined to react as little as possible.

The reading begins, and over the next twenty minutes, three people come through. I have no idea who they are. Karissa assures me that they're definitely for me, that "spirit doesn't make mistakes," and that I may well recognize them later, "which is common," she says.

"Okay," I say, envisioning a crowd of Disney-like hologram spirits elbowing each other aside to clamor around her.

Whoever they are—a musician I met in college, maybe? A great-aunt who died when I was young?—the messages do in fact resonate. They all refer to caretaking I did and they say that I am recovering and at a reset point in my life.

Still, I am disappointed.

Karissa at this point says that if I am really intent on having one person come through, I can tell her how I'm connected to the person, or give her a first name and she can ask everyone else to gently step back. It's up to me, she says, because otherwise she might keep getting these spirits she calls "icebreakers."

Okay. "My daughter," I say.

She tells me that as soon as I spoke, she saw everyone step back and Caitlin's energy connected, and Caitlin said, "The caretaking she did was for me."

For the next few minutes, the messages coming through from "Caitlin" are that she is happy and full of joy, that she did not feel fear when passing, that she wants to say thank you, that she feels my love, that we were not a typical mother-daughter pair.

The messages fit, but in a general way. Karissa asks if May is significant, and it is—it's my birthday month—but I'm thinking that May would be significant for any mother because of Mother's Day.

I glance down at my phone, which is recording the session. I'm thinking, *Now what?* There is no other way for me to try to communicate with my daughter, if indeed that is even possible, and it likely isn't, and I'm sitting here like the vulnerable grieving parent that I am.

"So she keeps wanting to talk to me about her hair," Karissa says. I snap my head up but Karissa's gaze is inward-focused.

"So I don't know if she had some massive hair change at the end, but she keeps showing me that her hair is silky and longer again and she's excited about this and wants me to tell you."

"Okay."

"And I keep coming back here to the sense that you relate to each other not as mother and daughter but as on the same page. Like as sisters." She says that we had a rare closeness and an ability to really talk to each other. "She's saying, 'I could talk to my mom about everything even if I didn't always.'" Karissa laughs. "She's telling me that having this relationship was a huge piece of her soul's path here. And that you gave her that true sense of unconditional love and she needs you to know that she felt that."

"Okay."

"She wants me to back up. Again, you did not make her feel like a burden. She's showing me that you would use humor, and I keep seeing a washcloth brought up to her face, and she's showing me that I feel like you had to care for her, toward the end, as you cared for her in the beginning of her life, and she's saying, 'I came full circle for you' and she wants to thank you for that love. She keeps saying, 'You did everything you could for me, you know this.'"

Karissa looks directly at me now. "Are you holding on to guilt or something? Because she's saying 'you have to let her know' that there's nothing more you could have done."

"Okay," I say, determined to be noncommittal.

"She's showing me that you feel frustrated that you're not getting signs or communication from her in a certain way. Do you understand that?"

"Yes. I feel like I'm feeling too desperate. And so I doubt everything."

"She's showing me, 'Just don't worry. I'm here, I'm coming to you, and I'm going to keep coming to you.' She keeps showing me trying to get to you through your dreams."

"I have not been able to remember my dreams."

"What I usually see happening and what she's acknowledging is that's just your grief. It's still covering and clouding them."

Her gaze shifts away again. "Now she's taking me backward. There's something about toward the end for her, where she feels really out of sorts and like she has no control over any of what's happening. And she's saying, 'I want you to go back over several years' and that's where she's showing me she is. She's telling you, 'I'm back there now.'"

Karissa hesitates a moment. "She's saying use this word lightly with my mother, but I want to acknowledge that there was physical suffering for her toward the end, and so the release to be free of that is huge for her soul and she wants to say, 'I'm very happy to not be in that body anymore.' So as much as she didn't want to leave anybody here, she wants to show her relief. She's also telling me, 'You were my anchor.' You were everything for her. She knows everything you did from the moment she was born. Is she your only daughter?"

"Yes."

"She's saying, 'I changed everything when I came into her life.' I feel like she was very unexpected for you. And she says, 'When I came, she was just kind of like oh no what am I going to do?' but it's like something clicked in you and everything you did after that was for her.

"She's funny," Karissa says. "She's witty. She's saying since she passed—she's making me feel like this is pretty recent, and you haven't had a moment yet to come down. She's saying you did the absolute best job that anyone could do and you haven't let yourself feel that, because I think that in your mind, losing her feels like you failed somehow. Also, she's showing me the month of December as being very significant. Do you understand that?"

"Yes."

"So this is only a matter of months that she's been passed, and she says will you give yourself some credit? In the sense of just sitting in this office to make this connection for the first time is a huge deal. So she's saying 'please give yourself some credit, Mom, and don't expect everything to be exactly how you wanted it or expected it to be.' This is such a close, close passing.

"She keeps showing me being at—not just the beach, but big big waves. Did she love to be in the water?"

"She loved the ocean."

"These are big. She's showing me big waves. Feels more like California ocean. I get the sense that she wanted to do a lot of traveling but it got cut short. And she's telling me, 'I'm doing that traveling now.' In spirit they can choose where they want to spend their time."

I decide to just go with all this. "Like where is she?"

"It's hard to say that they're omnipresent, but time is not in their reality. They have the ability to be with us and also be having these experiences, which we imagine as human-like but are created by their wants. Does that make sense?"

"We went to California after her service to see the big coastline."

"So it's significant for her to bring that through. She's saying, 'My poor mom, she's waiting to have this "experience" with me.' She's saying, 'Trust me, it's coming, not in the way you think it is, it's never going to be on your timeline.'"

Karissa is quiet for a few long moments. "It's funny," she says, "I do feel like she's sending you tons of signs, but I just don't know if you're aware to look for them."

"No," I say. "I think I am getting tons of signs, but I just doubt them all. But I get them all the time."

Karissa laughs, and says that Caitlin is laughing, too, and saying, "'Mom, what's it going to take for you to feel like this is real?' I think this is the last thing you'd ever expect to hear her say, but she's saying, 'Faith is a choice.'"

I think about that. I have always associated the word "faith" with organized religion, with beliefs that others try to impose on me, but of course faith is any belief not based on proof. Faith is confidence. It is trust.

Karissa addresses me directly now and advises me not to put so much pressure on myself. "Knowing these signs are coming from her is going to take time."

Knowing. Knowing means certainty. I know what knowing feels like, and this doesn't feel like knowing.

"She's saying, 'My mom's the last person I thought would struggle with this.'

"Since she passed," she says, "did you have a minor scuffle in your car? It's funny that she used the words 'minor scuffle.' I'm not feeling like it's an accident here, but something that happened and could have been a lot worse."

"No," I say, although the word "scuffle" is such a Caitlin word. But no, I have a long, clean driving record. I haven't had any "scuffles."

Karissa looks skeptical. "I don't know how your memory is right now but just take that with you and see if you remember something. She's saying, 'minor scuffle but could have been a lot worse and it just kind of sorted itself out.' She's saying that was her energy and she just wants that to be known."

It's only later, as I listen to the recording and type up the transcript, that I remember one day in January. I had been crying and inattentive and I jerked the wheel too hard as I drove out of our driveway. I smashed into our front stone wall and knocked down a large portion of it.

Karissa moves on. "She keeps showing me that she was either a talented writer or that she left writing behind. Do you understand that? She's telling me that it was very important and she wants it to be heralded. Her writings are the musings of her soul, and in those pieces—key pieces that are your favorites—when you read these, you can feel her essence there."

"Okay."

"She's saying that she loved that you didn't have expectations for her, that you completely let her be who she was. She's saying you have a feminist heart, and I feel like you're very intelligent, too. She keeps pointing to your brain, so are you very well read?"

"I like to read."

"She's saying, 'She's very well read and intelligent and she gave me those feminist musings and a backbone and I fought for myself, she gave me no feminine archetypal expectations, she let me be whoever I wanted to be and that is a freedom that is so not afforded to so many people.' And she's grateful."

Karissa shifts gears again. "Okay, now she's saying, 'I want to focus on you now.'"

"Me?"

"She's saying, 'Mom, everybody's been saying it right to you, this is a reset. That's what it is. It's not a reset you want. But it's one that you have to deal with anyway.' I keep seeing you walking outside and being in nature, having quiet times in spring. And she's telling me that this is going to be really healing and it's those quiet times by yourself that you're really going to feel like you're connecting with her."

"She's saying, 'My mom is also a really talented writer' and now she's showing me 'author' and saying you could write a book about the loss that you experienced with her. She's showing me that you have this ability and sharing your story and sharing the loss of her would be very beneficial for you and would also be very healing to many other people. Have you written about it at all, like journaling?"

"I've been keeping a blog."

"Okay. Perfect. I don't know if you've considered writing a book but she's showing me you're going to do this, that it's definitely happening."

I'm still sitting as expressionless as possible, trying not to show that I do now feel like Caitlin might just be in this space with us.

Karissa says, "Nobody who loses a child is ready to let them go, but this is different in that you're having your belief system challenged in every single way, at the same time. She's saying that these are the themes that need to be brought through in your book."

"She's also showing me that you do art, or that you are connected very artistically. Do you do any drawing or painting?"

"No."

"She's showing you mixing colors, that you have an artist's soul."

"I've often written about artists."

"It's like she's trying to put the paints in your hand."

Karissa talks about how I am a perfectionist, then shifts. "She wants to speak about herself again. She's showing me some kind of a foundation that you're starting for her, do you understand that? In her name. As you move forward. I feel like it's not in the works yet but it's coming. Does that make sense?"

I think about my idea for a portable healing garden, which I have been turning over and over in my mind. I visualize a vehicle fitted out like something secret and magical, with space for swappable garden elements. But so many sick people, like Caitlin herself, cannot be around flowers, plants, dirt. Perhaps a sound garden, of sorts, a garden of music . . .

"Okay," I say.

"Okay." Karissa looks at me with some concern. "I'm just checking in with you. How is this communication working for you? Are you okay with this?"

She's kind and concerned and I know I sound rude but I want to remain noncommittal. I say, "Yes."

"I want to make sure this is resonating with you."

"Yes, I can imagine you would." Ouch. Rude.

"Well, it's a very recent loss, and those can often be the most difficult to bring through. Does that make sense?"

I say that it does. And that I didn't even know if it was time yet.

"Caitlin's ready," she says. "It's our grief that gets in the way."

Karissa moves on. "She keeps also showing me that she's very music-oriented. She's saying, 'I'm trying to send my mom music but she didn't always like the same things that I listened to.' But she's very music-oriented and she's wanting to bring through speaking to you through music as well, she's saying, 'Just keep paying attention.' Now, going back in time, she makes me feel like you love—I feel like there's shared undertones of music that she grew up with you. Did you listen to Joni Mitchell? She keeps saying, 'Listen to Joni Mitchell.'"

For the first time in this session, I freeze. I'm reminded of the day Caitlin and I saw that medium John Holland, when it felt like my father briefly inhabited John's body and Caitlin dug her nails into mine.

"Joni Mitchell?"

"Yeah. Or something of this era, maybe?"

"*She* loved Joni Mitchell." I am trying to emphasize that Caitlin was the Joni lover, not me. "*Loved* her."

"She's saying, 'Let me speak to you in Joni.'"

Karissa doesn't realize that this Joni reference has rocked me. She talks about how music can be an express pathway to Caitlin, "more important than any words anyone's going to say to you." She talks about how even when she was little, Caitlin had a mind of her own and was unconventional, and didn't hold back and that she owed that to me.

"Grief is the most deafening sense of loneliness that can come over anybody. And she says that really, death is quite the opposite, there's a sense of unity and a sense of wholeness."

Karissa laughs abruptly. "She says, 'There was no tunnel, by the way!'"

I'm staring at her now, watching this woman who is focused inwardly and communicating . . . with my deceased daughter?

"She keeps making me feel like you really want to know how her passing was."

"I do, actually," I say, but I'm thinking, *Is this real? Can she really tell me? No one could make this up. Only a cruel person would try.*

"Everybody has a different experience is what I've learned as a medium. But she keeps coming through, like, 'You know, Mom, I just closed my eyes and woke up somewhere else. It really was as simple as I kind of fluttered my eyes and then it was "Hmm, what is this place?" It was all of a sudden, just being in a different place, it wasn't like this strange sense of "sucked up" or anything like that,' and she's showing me it was actually quite wonderful, that she was met by all of this beautiful energy and she's like—again, I feel like she had some beliefs but she wasn't sure what to believe, either—'so I kind of had to look and think, "Oh, is this that thing?" And then it was.'"

"That thing." Speaking "in Joni." These are Caitlin phrases. Just as "damn good concert" and "got the green light" had sounded like Caitlin in Shelley's reading with Sirrý.

"I feel like for her it was very much a sense of—'I'm here, and one moment I'm somewhere else.' So I feel like 'peace with that' is what she wants to show you. Like it not being this big process. Does that make sense?"

"Yes. I mean, of course I'm curious. But I have to wait and see for myself."

"Well, I suppose that's true. But she wants to give rest to your heart and say, 'Truly it's not a process. There's no big . . .' You know, we think it's going to be this tidal wave of an experience, and she's like, 'No, it's just this sense of all of a sudden you've got no physical limitations or pain. It's this pure sense of freedom that comes through.'"

"Okay."

Karissa turns focused and serious. "Okay, so she wants to come back and take me to right before she passes."

I sit very still. No one could Google this, or make this up.

"Okay, she wants me to acknowledge you on her left side of her body. And she wants to say that you acknowledged to her that it was okay to go." She pauses, laughs softly. "Even though you didn't mean it. And she laughs with me, saying, 'That's my mom, doing whatever she had to do to make me feel better even if it wasn't true.'"

I'm quiet, processing this, but I am starting to simmer with something—excitement, wonder, curiosity.

The recording app is racing toward the hour mark and she says, "She wants me to give you tremendous amounts of love. And gratitude. You were the best mother that could ever have happened to her. She's funny. She says, 'I picked the right one.' And she says, 'Go back to yoga.' Did you used to do yoga? She's pushing me back there. You have to pick up on the self-care again. She's like, 'And I'm watching you.'"

I smile inwardly. Another Caitlin phrase.

"She's saying, 'This is the new dawn of you learning to live with me in a different way.' And that book is going to be about the two of you. It's not just your book, it's her book, too."

Karissa is winding up now. "Be patient with yourself," she says. "Grief is still very close. Let the information sit. They work with us where we are in the . . ."

The focusing look returns to her face. "Also, I just want to say that hawks are very strongly connected to her. She's been flashing me hawks. I forgot to say it, because I only get two-thirds out of my mouth that they want to push through. She keeps saying, 'I am the hawks.'"

I practically fall out of my chair then. I say, "Are you kidding?"

"She's trying so hard to be like, 'Here I am.' We talk about the veil? The veil is grief. As that lifts, then our communication with them lifts. Grief has its own timeline and all we can do is respect it."

I feel lighter after the reading. More hopeful. We plan a night for some of Caitlin's close friends to come to dinner. Instead of my usual jazz stations that I put on for parties, I decide to take the advice and speak in Joni.

I choose a Joni Mitchell station, but as I cook, I notice that the station is playing no Joni, and that the songs it is playing seem ridiculously message-like. I start jotting down the titles:

"Spirit in the Sky," Norman Greenbaum;
"Let's Live for Today," the Grass Roots;
"Turn, Turn, Turn—to Every Season," the Byrds;
"Stairway to Heaven," Led Zeppelin—aside from the obvious, we used to laugh because a volunteer harpist at the inpatient units at Brigham and Women's Hospital always played it and we'd think, *Um, not appropriate!!*;
"Last Dance with Mary Jane," Tom Petty—a lifelong elementary school inside joke;
"The Sound of Silence," Simon & Garfunkel.

Finally, a Joni song comes on, one I don't know. At first I think I am not hearing correctly and check the info screen. "Willy," Joni Mitchell. Nick's younger brother Willie died when Caitlin was five. Caitlin adored him. Willie was Caitlin's first experience with death.

The friends arrive, and someone says, "Hey! This sounds like Caitlin's music!" I mention how the music has been a bit spooky and message-like, and as I talk, I realize what is playing. I can't believe it. I say, "I can't believe this."

I run upstairs to get the little notebook I found in January, the one with the word LIFE on its cover, and I pass it around.

You can't always get what you want, and if you try sometimes, you get what you need.

Let go. Just be strong. You will not be able to predict the future. Accept that. You are getting what you need.

But it is going to be scary and you might die.

God.

❧

I often drive through the cemetery but I have only been inside the mausoleum once. The mausoleum is a cold and creepy crypt and I will be happy when we have built our private one. But on the day after the dinner party, I'm compelled to go in.

I'd looked forward to the dinner and had loved it but now that it's over, I feel Caitlin's absence even more keenly.

Inside, I start to quake and cry at the thought that *she is really right there on the other side of that wall*. I knock on the marble and speak. *Where are you, buddy? Where are you? How can you really be in there?*

After a moment, I step away to wipe my eyes, and realize something. Her space is adjacent to someone whose last name was PARIS and whose first name was BIRDIE.

Really? Birdie Paris? I stop crying and look around the cold, silent chamber. Is she here? Watching? Laughing at the sight of me finally noticing this coincidence?

Back in my car, I text a few people to tell them. I write, *Come on!!! Birdie Paris??*

And as I pull out of the cemetery and merge onto the road, the car in front of me bears a bumper sticker that reads, *Meow!*

You really can't make this stuff up.

⁂

Jess, my sister, and I travel to London to spend a little time with Sinéad. We visit the Chelsea Physic Garden, a place Caitlin discovered and loved, which the Worshipful Society of Apothecaries established in 1673 to grow plants for medicines.

I talk to myself there. *See? Modern medicine is still so new. It is, compared to the wonder that is the human body itself, actually still quite primitive. You were lucky to have had a CF child for thirty-three years, to have lived in the first century where children weren't expected to die.*

And thoughts like that make you feel better in the moment, but then it is May, it is Mother's Day, and people are kind and attentive, Caitlin's friends gather around, and you are so grateful for what you had and still have but there is nothing to be done about the pain that persists.

14

THE SOUND OF SILENCE

I am not the first person to compare time to a river, but from my desk overlooking the water, the comparison is ever present, the imagery apt. Drop something into the river and off it goes. It's never coming back.

It's six months today. And a Tuesday, just as it was then. Late June. Another solstice.

And the great world spins.

We lost Caitlin in winter and because winter lasted forever, time felt elastic, a time in which she still existed, was still somewhat "of the present." Now New England has done its thing and jumped from raw/rainy/nasty/cold to suddenly summer. A new season that emphasizes the finality of her absence. Yet every day we still experience the jolt: it can't be true. Disbelief accompanied by images of her face, her voice, her presence, despair.

The season starts with unusual but welcome visitors. Erin, Caitlin's ICU nurse, is first. She arrives with her husband and three little daughters. In July, Penny spends a week in Caitlin's apartment with her mother and daughter as they tour Boston.

Plenty of people found these visits unusual and worried that they would be too painful for us. *We* worried. But they weren't. Our time in the ICU wasn't normal human time. Erin and Penny were there for the most dramatic days of our lives. They tried to save Caitlin. We forged a strong bond. Erin tells me that Caitlin changed her life, that she considers her to be a kind of guide.

Their visits give me the courage to email Larry, Caitlin's transplant coordinator, to start to deal with things. I want the films of her native lungs, want to see what she had to breathe with all those years. I want to know where to write a thank-you note to the donor family.

He sends the films, but it will be months before I can open the file and look at them.

I'm so glad to hear from you. I saw Erin and she said you were going to email me. How are you and Nick doing? I hope every day continues to ease the pain. I think about both of you often, in fact, I don't know if you were aware of this, but there is an O'Hara street that runs right into the hospital. I've been holding on to this one as well . . . for three evenings immediately after Caitlin passed the birds kept flying overheard. I mean whole hordes of them, no exaggeration, there must have been a few thousand as far as I could see, all flying in a flowing wave. I've never seen anything like it. Quite incredible.

People continue to send messages, letters, cat- and bird-themed gifts, and now, heart-shaped rocks for the mausoleum.

In our kitchen window, I've hung two of the bird ornaments. One is a small metal bluebird gifted to me by my Pittsburgh friend Jane. The other is a ceramic blue jay from my Vertex friend Patrick.

One morning in July, Nick opens one of the windows and the ceramic blue jay drops onto the floor and breaks into three pieces. He rarely yells, but he does now. "Damn it! That's why I don't like things hanging on these windows!" And I yell back, "Well, you just have to be careful!"

But our yelling ends abruptly as a real bird appears on the other side of the window, hover-fluttering in place, just looking in at us. We gape at it. We've never seen a bird do that. When it finally flies away, we look at each other.

We've been married a long time and we've been through a lot. No sense messing it up. We realize we can fix the bird with Super Glue, and do. Good as new. I hang it in a dining room window that we never open.

Later, I put on one of Caitlin's playlists, even though the first song on the playlist is Bob Seger's "Roll Me Away," which I've been afraid to hear because it will remind me of how Caitlin played it while I ran, pushing her wheelchair to the fast beat, both of us laughing, through a deserted hospital corridor on one of those first November nights when she still felt normal and transplant seemed finally, joyously imminent.

I am puttering around the kitchen and sort of listening to the lyrics. Then I do a double take and restart the song. Seger is singing about being alone with choices and about his soul rising and his heart singing at the sight of a young hawk. And those lyrics feel very fitting in that moment. They really do.

❦

We are on Martha's Vineyard to host a celebration of Caitlin's July thirty-first birthday with her close friends and all I can think about is how crushingly relieved, how full of joy I would have been if someone had told us, last summer, that Caitlin would get her transplant and that we would be celebrating her next birthday on the Vineyard.

The Vineyard was Caitlin's place. She recovered here after her months in the hospital when she was eleven, and we often rented for a week or two each summer. And for years, she and Jess and their friend Liz visited Jess's mom's house in Chilmark for restorative weekends. "We don't party," Caitlin would report. "We drink milk, eat pie, go to the beach, and sleep."

This time, we are renting a house I found as if by divine intervention. It is named LovingKindness Retreat, and it is owned by an angel of a woman who generally rents to Buddhist monks on retreat, or yogis. This is the first time she has rented to the general public.

The house is clean and airy, with a simple white color theme. The backyard gardens are full of birds. A welcoming note sits on the kitchen counter, as well as a treat for Henry.

We arrange big, laminated prints of Caitlin around the house, and these images surround us at the gathering, which is fun and lively. We love Caitlin's friends, and luckily they love us. After the barbecue, I give everyone a small island-made berry pie, each adorned with a golden, glittery candle. I ask people to light their candles and to take a mindful moment to wish for something good and happy for their own souls.

Then Andrew passes out sparklers. We light them outside and dedicate them to Caitlin.

Later, I am struck to see how normal Nick and I look in all the photos. Happy faces, big smiles. Photographs lie more than I ever realized.

I am still on the island and I go for a drive. At 7A, a busy little farm-to-takeout shop that Caitlin loved and talked about all winter, obsessed with their local sausage biscuit sandwiches, I buy a coffee and get back in my car. The parking lot is crowded and other cars hover, waiting for open spots. A trio of tall, healthy-looking young women stroll past me, eating ice cream and laughing. As I back out of my spot I start to cry, and talk aloud to Caitlin. "I wish you could have had good health like that," I say.

I have to wait to let a car back out in front of me. License plate 333.

A sign, another one, but they never seem to be enough, only helping for the brief moment it takes me to register them.

I decide to drive out to the far end of the island, down Lobsterville Road, a skinny stretch of pavement that follows the curving peninsula of Lobsterville Beach, to reenact the last time we were on-island and Caitlin and I drove all the way out there. Even in the height of summer, it's a part of the island where you rarely see other people, just long, empty stretches of beach open only to residents. Houses are few.

I decide to go all the way to the end, as I had with Caitlin that day, where the road ends at a small turn-around and boat ramp.

As I drive, I am saying things aloud. "What the heck?? Why does it have to be this way? Why can't we communicate if you're really out there?"

I try to remind myself of Karissa, and the hawks, and speak to me in Joni, but I'm jammed inside Earth's physical plane, and today is one of those days when a tangible afterlife is fantasy.

She's gone, I think. *There's nothing else. I will never see her again.*

"I loved you from the first minute," I say, and I am crying now. "No one will ever call me 'Mom' again."

I turn into the dead-end area where the road stops at the water and I pass him: a guy who is all by himself out there, carrying a burlap bag with three big red letters on its side, an acronym for something. Three red letters that spell MOM.

"You look much better than the last time I saw you," says a friend I haven't seen in months.

Really? How can that be? I am a leaf caught in a current and I have no control over that current. I spin within eddies, I drown and revive, and sometimes I float, eyes fixed on the sky.

When I leave my friend and walk through the hot Boston streets, I look more closely at the chatting faces, the heads bent to phones, the moving mouths, the smiles, the frowns, the blank expressions, and wonder what's behind each one.

How hard it is to tell anything, really, about a person from the outside.

What am I waiting for?

Assurance. Clarity. *Knowing*.

But I am inside Plato's cave, watching a show of shadows and wondering what is real. There's no denying that strange synchronicities have happened and keep happening, so many more than I can recount here. To insist they are not meaningful, to discount them, seems almost myopic.

Sinéad is in touch with me almost daily, by text. She receives her own clear messages. Sinéad has no doubt, but she sees, hears, and *knows* in a way I can't.

Did Caitlin have her own version of knowing what was to

come? *I've always thought I was going to die of a stroke*, she'd said. *I am so terrified of having a stroke like that. Locked-in syndrome. I am so so afraid of it in ways I can't even be ok with.*

What a mystery is this existence of ours.

When Nick's brother Willie died of an aneurysm, here in the United States, his mother, who still had eight living children, tamped down her once-adventurous spirit. She never again visited us in the United States, because she was afraid it would be too painful. Even though it must have also been painful not to visit her son and only American grandchild.

Nick and I are aware that we don't want to cut ourselves off from the family experiences we always loved, and so in September, we start to think about St. John.

I begin looking for a small villa for the two of us. We'll stay in that for half the time, and half the time at Caneel Bay, one of the only hotels on the little island.

I've just begun my villa search when hurricane warnings start. Then Irma hits, and a week later, Maria. Two category 5 hurricanes tearing through the islands, sucking away every bit of vegetation.

A couple of restaurants we'd been visiting since the 1990s? Flattened. Gone. Our favorite villa, Spellbound, the one I'd had to cancel when Caitlin got sick? Destroyed, its roof blown off. Caneel Bay closed, with no opening date in sight.

There is no going back to what was. That old human lesson.

Onward, life is saying. *Onward.* And my feet feel for that onward path but can't yet find it.

My sister's daughter Jillian is getting married. A September wedding in coastal Maine. We are staying at a resort in Rockland that is, strangely, less than a mile from the home of the astrologer who gave me that reading Caitlin gifted me with in 2015.

I decide I want to see her. I book an appointment for the day before the wedding. As dire as part of that reading had been (after I had, to be fair, pushed twice for clarification), it had been accurate. Maybe she can tell me something that will shine light on the mysteries.

There's anger in my chart, she tells me.

"Oh, I don't feel anger," I say. "What good is anger? Anger changes nothing. Anger would only make me feel worse."

"Well," she says, "you can rationalize it all you want, but anger is there and maybe you'd better express it."

Jillian's wedding is lovely and Jillian is lovely and she has thoughtfully placed a heart-shaped frame containing a photograph of Caitlin at our table, but there is pain to know that Caitlin will never have the small, private ceremony she wanted, in Tuscany perhaps, where she had found a rental villa that looked clean and airy and bright and good for new lungs, its name fortuitous. Villa Lungomonte. There will never be the little daughter she might have adopted or had by surrogate, whom she would have named Joni.

The morning after the wedding, I log on to Facebook, and the first thing in my feed is Dr. D'Cunha's face. He is wearing his blue surgical cap and white coat and he is posing with Mallory, who is sitting up in the familiar hospital bed, both of them wearing big smiles.

After three dry runs, Mallory has been called to transplant, and this fourth offer looks good. This date also marks the tenth anniversary of the successful transplant of Caitlin's friend Meg, the one who also had cepacia and was transplanted in Boston before the rules changed.

Outside our hotel, a mile-long stone pier leads to a lighthouse. Nick and I walk it, and at the end, where we find ourselves alone with the stone and the water and the wind, I scream and scream.

⁂

September 18 is our wedding anniversary, and nine months since the lung transplant on December 18.

Nine months.

Let's walk around Walden Pond, I suggest, and we drive the short distance to Concord. As we follow the meandering, wooded path that circles the tranquil pond, I tell Nick I am putting pressure on myself to figure out the puzzle of the portable healing garden. If sick people can't breathe plants and dirt, would it make sense to separate the garden elements with glass walls? Make the garden a feast for at least one of the senses? Or maybe it could be a sound garden? With music? Oliver Sacks wrote that in forty years of medical practice, he found only two types of nonpharmaceutical therapy to be vitally important for patients with chronic neurological diseases: music and gardens.

Nick tells me that the garden will come, in time. That we don't have to do everything right this minute. We'll figure it out, he says.

I've known Nick since I was twenty years old. We've grown up together. Our relationship has had its unsteady moments, like many, but we share the same values and we balance each other. I'm hyperconscious, now, of the fact that we are getting older and that one of us likely will go before the other and that statistics say it will likely be him. I try to live in the moment, appreciate what I have, remember that nothing is forever.

I think about Thoreau in these woods, and the other nineteenth-century writers. Walt Whitman was one of Caitlin's favorites from a precociously early age, and he is in my head. *Not in another place, but this place. Not for another hour, but this hour. These are the days that must happen to you.*

I think of my hours these past months, my leaf life.

Reset. Rebirth. After months of doing very little, I decide I am going to begin to rouse myself a bit. I decide I will do two things every day: I will meditate, and I will write a book about Caitlin. And maybe that will help me find my path.

Through a friend, I meet a clairvoyant and meditation teacher at a party, a woman whose new book has just been published by Penguin. Her name is Ellen Tadd. She is tall, conservatively dressed, and interacts with such a calm, serious demeanor that she seems more like a research scientist or university professor. At one point she mentions that her father had been a physicist, and I wonder if she drops that information frequently, to help retract skeptical antennae.

If so, it works. It retracts mine. She is credible. We discover we have a mutual friend, an editor whom I greatly respect. We talk easily.

I tell her about Caitlin, and her response is not the sympathetic one I've become accustomed to.

Death, she says, is like one person going into another room and shutting the door. "You're here, they're on the other side," she says. "That's all it is."

Like Sinéad, she has no doubts. She *knows*.

I read her new book and am particularly drawn to what she calls "I am spirit" consciousness. I adapt her words to make my own for inclusion in my daily meditation practice.

I am spirit.
Caitlin is spirit.
I am temporarily human.
Caitlin was temporarily human.
We are all spirit.
We are all temporarily human.

On the blog, I announce that I will be writing fewer posts because I am going to write a book about "all this." A writer friend asks whether I have ever considered attending one of Dani Shapiro's occasional, women-only, memoir-writing retreats.

I didn't know about them, but I'm still a leaf in a current and so I write to Dani. She responds with a spot for me, if I want it, in November.

Over the years, I've read Dani's work in *The New Yorker* and remember a compelling essay, "Plane Crash Theory," that we published in *Ploughshares* during my time there. Now I read one of her newer books, *Devotion*, a beautiful, achingly spare memoir about one person's search for meaning, and think, *Yes, she seems the perfect influence for the beginning of this project.*

We will be seven writers in a Connecticut inn for two days and two nights. There will be yoga and meditation. Having a deadline, even if it is only ten pages, will be helpful, and get me into a focusing frame of mind.

When Dani sends me the address where I can send a check to pay for the retreat, I see that the post office box number is 33.

Does it mean something? As she writes in *Devotion*, quoting a conversation she had with a man who escaped the towers on 9/11, if something seems like it should mean something, "you make it mean something. That's all you can do."

❧

In late October, I am reading the pages of the other writers who will be at Dani's retreat. One of the names is nagging at me. It seems so familiar and I realize that Julie Himes is the author of the novel our book club is reading for December, a book that is lying on the table right beside me. I write to Julie to say hello and to remark on the coincidence.

She responds with a remarkable coincidence of her own. In my ten pages, I had mentioned Vertex Pharmaceuticals' Kalydeco, the gene-correcting cystic fibrosis drug that Patrick, the scientist who had written to me while we were in the hospital, coinvented and that might have indefinitely prolonged Caitlin's life if she'd had access to it before her extensive lung damage occurred. In addition to being a writer, the multitalented Julie is also a research physician and a medical director at Vertex.

Another interesting coincidence, and not one my antennae had much to do with. Does it mean something? I decide to make it mean I'm meant to write this story.

The retreat turns out to be both grounding and inspiring, with meditation and yoga and good conversation. As I am leaving, Dani suggests I come to the writing workshop that she and her husband run in Positano, Italy, the week before Easter every year.

Caitlin's health was always so precarious that even when CF was in the box, I was always poised to cancel all plans when a cleanout became necessary. I never applied to residencies or attended conferences or planned much that required any kind of advance decision.

But now I can do whatever I want, so I take her advice.

It will be good to have a purpose, a goal—twenty-five pages of this book, to submit to the workshop by early February.

&

I observe Mallory's posttransplant milestones via texts from her mother and from Mary and Ralph. Mallory's has been a tougher than normal recovery but she is eventually discharged and continues to improve.

One day, Mallory's mother reports that Mallory walked forty-seven hundred steps and that the final two drains and remaining staples had been removed from her surgical site. Exuberant Mallory had exclaimed, "Today is the best day of my life!"

Mallory celebrates her twenty-fifth birthday in October and is beginning to dare to imagine the life she's been gifted. She wants to get home to California and live on the beach with her boyfriend, wants to work on the memoir she has been writing since she was a teen.

And then two months after her transplant, a pneumonia takes sudden, vicious hold and proves difficult to treat because of the nature of her cepacia, still colonized in her upper airways, and the immunosuppressants she must take.

Her father, a brilliant man who has long suspected that something called *phage therapy*, whereby a phage—a virus that destroys cells—can be matched to and then selectively isolated to kill specific bacteria, contacts Dr. Steffanie Strathdee, a Canadian epidemiologist who recently used phage therapy to save her own husband from a superbug infection. Dr. Strathdee sends out a plea across the planet to other phage researchers, and in a race against time, labs seek to match phages to Mallory's bacterial cultures.

Labs match two phages and rush them to Pittsburgh, but the

attempt at treatment comes too late for Mallory, and Mallory Smith becomes another example of how the very, very good—the ones who have so much to teach us—seem to be the ones who die so very, very young.

⁂

November 20. Another twentieth. Time moves forward forever, and Caitlin is receding into the forever past, and that cracks my heart.

On this evening I try to distract myself with cooking. I am chopping apricots and vegetables for a Moroccan tagine, listening to Erik Satie on Sonos, my eyes so full of tears that the onions have become a blurry pile of white.

I miss her I miss her I miss her. I can't believe it. Can't. If disbelief is a stage of grief, then I'm stuck in it. Because how can it really be true? And what is this life for, really? If souls don't exist and endure, then what the hell is the point? How can I keep going?

I hear what Caitlin might say. "Jeeeeez, Mame. You can start by turning off that depressing music. Why don't you try talking in Joni?"

Was that even true? The medium's message? Or was it some mind-boggling ability to read my mind? Does it matter? It was something Caitlin would definitely say. So I dry my eyes. I switch to the Joni Mitchell station and I'm struck, not for the first time, by Joni's self-awareness, her ability to articulate the complicated reality of being a human being, alive in a complicated world.

When the tagine is assembled and simmering, I go outside to get some fresh air and check the mail. There is a parcel from a name I recognize, a woman who has commented on the blog.

Inside the package is a small blue ceramic bird. A small box containing heart-shaped rocks. An iPod containing "playlists inspired by Caitlin." And a letter. *You don't know me but . . .*

December 20. A year. An impossible year.

I come awake. It's dark. I'm thinking of Andrew, and how he was the one on watch a year ago right now. I slip out of bed and open my phone. It's five twenty-three and Andrew has just texted a heart.

ANDREW: ❤

MARYANNE: Just JUST woke up thinking of you!

MARYANNE: ♥

ANDREW: I'm usually not up this early. It was weird, I was having a dream. Something entered it and just cancelled what was happening. Wide awake with 12/20 on the mind

MARYANNE: Caitlin must have woken us up at the same time

ANDREW: I think so!

MARYANNE: I was literally thinking of how you were on watch, last year at that time

ANDREW: I was thinking the same. Shift ended early morning

MARYANNE: Yes. All was stable

From: Caitlin O'Hara
To: A friend with CF who had a successful lung transplant
Date: July 8, 2016
Subject: Station Eleven

I keep thinking of you because I finally started Station Eleven. I knew it was supposed to be great, but once I read it was kind of about the flu I was like, "Eehh maybe I shouldn't read it" . . . Then when I saw that you loved it I thought, OK, she is just as paranoid as me so it can't really be that bad. I am about 100 pages in and totally hooked. Anyway it's really not about the flu in a "contagion" type sense, as I am seeing now, so I'm fine with it. But parts of the book made me choke up even right in the beginning. When she is describing what the world is like after the collapse. All the little things. That part, I just grabbed my book and looked it up, Chapter 6, "an incomplete list"—that small list of things just made me shiver with how MUCH this world is, all the small delights. And I loved how she used so many things that are the marvels of the modern world, and not just the generally accepted good things, but things like scrolling through social media, taking photographs of concerts, etc, because so much of what we read and hear today is about how all of that is bad bad, too much technology, too much noise, too much too much . . . when really there is SO MUCH magic to it. It's not all bad, of course. I would not know you were if not for the wonders of little screens and invisible connections through space. I also love how the book is not just a typical "dystopia" where everyone is some kind of rebel fighter that has survived. It feels real, and leaves so much to think about living in an old Wendy's or using old Snapple bottles . . . what would become useful, and how, and what would really be LOST.

15

SPEAK TO ME IN JONI

CAITLIN: Success after transplant is not a guarantee, it is something that comes with doing things right. There are a lot of interesting things in here about food safety, some that even I didn't know.

CAITLIN: After transplant, you guys are going to have to be way more vigilant than you are right now. You think this is tough?

CAITLIN: I ordered this book called Pittsburgh Steps and after transplant, I'm going to climb all the steps.

CAITLIN: Alcohol and Purell don't kill C diff—which I didn't know—hand washing only does—so important to keep in mind. Perhaps have a talking to with Daddy and Andrew about that. They just love to Purell and think they're all super clean. Not so. Important now and after transplant.

CAITLIN: I wrote to this shelter that has cats and asked them if I could come play with them. This is what I wrote: I love cats, but as it is cannot live with them because of my compromised lungs (too much hair and dander for daily living). I really want to play with some kittens, and in general just visit with some animals before my transplant. Would that be something you would allow? For me to just come in and meet them and play with them? I am sorry I won't be able to adopt one, but I am more than happy to make a donation and try to spread the word about any animals that need adopting!

CAITLIN: I dreamed it was after transplant and I was running.

CAITLIN: After transplant, we can go to Paris. Paris for every Mother's Day!

We are in Sausalito and it is exactly one year since we sought shelter here last January. We are even in the same hotel room, which is the ground floor of a historic house in what was once a military fort at the base of the Golden Gate Bridge.

I think I was seeking comfort, coming back here. Our grief was so fresh last year. Caitlin felt "with us." But when I see the laminated photograph of her on the fireplace mantel, exactly where Nick placed it last year, it feels all wrong.

The night before we flew here, as I was driving into Boston, the songs that came on the radio were dark, reminders of mortality. I drove past the cemetery just as The Doors' "The End" came on. Then Queen, "Tie Your Mother Down," which I never hear on the radio. Brian May wrote it and acknowledges that the title really has no meaning, but as it began to play, a hawk whizzed across the turnpike, right in front of my windshield, so close I jerked the wheel and yelped.

A few minutes later, I realized I was behind a hearse, and Steely Dan was singing about California tumbling into the sea.

Our first night in San Francisco, the chatter of an earthquake wakes me up. The next morning, driving the winding road along the Marin Headlands, another hawk flies at our window.

In our hotel gym, the attendant reaches into a basket of locker keys and hands me one. I see it is number thirty-four. *Too bad it isn't thirty-three*, I think. But as I fit it into the locker, I think, *No, it's right that it's thirty-four. Caitlin would be thirty-four now.* Another reminder that time moves forward on this planet.

As part of this Groundhog Day trip, we stay in Big Sur again.

On our last night, we decide to have dinner at a tiny restaurant called Big Sur Bakery. The maître d' is a warm, charming native of Spain and France who spends a few moments speaking with Nick before seating us in a corner of the dining room. The room is cozy, glowing with reddish light from the fireplace.

We have ordered and are talking about our day when I see Nick's face change, become disbelieving.

"What is it?" I turn to look. A young man is pushing a young woman in a wheelchair into the restaurant. The young woman is wearing oxygen. If I were to squint my eyes, the two could be Andrew and Caitlin.

Nick and I just look at each other in disbelief. Big Sur is an isolated part of a rugged coastal peninsula of steep cliffs and redwoods. It has a population of eight hundred and is hours from the major medical centers. What are they doing here?

From where Nick sits, he has a clear view to where the maître d' seats them. Nick doesn't realize that it is obvious he's having an emotional time. At one point, the maître d' comes over and puts his hands on Nick's shoulders and says, "You are a good man. I can tell this."

Nick is confused. He still doesn't realize that his pain is all over his face. I try to tell him but he's completely discombobulated. We eat our dinners, hyperaware, the entire time, of the couple who eat super quickly and soon rise to leave.

I think of how most people would avoid looking at Caitlin's oxygen and wheelchair, out of politeness, and how it could make her feel invisible. I decide I will just say a warm hello as they pass, but somehow Nick and I both say hi and Nick asks her if she has CF, and at the same time I say, "So does our daughter."

Her face brightens. "How old is she?"

"Thirty-three, and she had a transplant and it went really well." Because I can't tell her and anyway, why not give someone the hope we had? But I don't want her to follow up so I keep talking. "And not only that, her friend just celebrated her tenth transplant anniversary and she's doing great and how old are you?"

"Twenty-five."

"I take it you are listed."

"At UCLA."

"How long have you been waiting?"

"About a year. It will happen."

"How tall are you?"

"Five-one."

"What's your blood type?"

"I don't know."

"How much oxygen are you on?"

"Two liters."

She sounds so breathless. She needs more here. Does she know that? Even being here, twelve hundred feet above sea level, isn't wise.

"Thanks for saying hello," she says.

We watch them through the window, the familiar routines—

lifting the tanks, folding the wheelchair—still struck dumb by the strangeness of this coincidence.

"She didn't even know her blood type," Nick says. He is angry. "I want to tell her, tell her she needs to pay attention."

I point out that Caitlin controlled everything, but in the end, she'd had no control at all.

Nick sees the hawks and thirty-threes and all the other signs, too. He struggles with doubt less than I do. He takes comfort in the signs. He talks to Caitlin and says he really feels he is conversing.

"Maybe," I say, "seeing this girl was a kind message for us. A hello. A reminder not to be bitter, a reminder that everyone on this planet is on his or her own path."

⁂

Previously, when I thought about or met someone who had lost a child, I assumed that the passage of time helped. That someone, say, whose son died of cancer ten years ago was probably doing okay by now.

In Los Angeles, we see Mallory's parents. When Mallory's mother asks me if it gets better, my first thought is to say no. Then I realize that I no longer wake up each morning and have to remember everything all over again. So that particular agony has abated.

I've learned that it doesn't get better, I say. It just gets different.

⁂

In February, friends on St. John urge us to come down. The island is getting back on its feet, they say. The beaches are still beautiful, restaurants are open. The island needs visitors.

So we fly in and the pain of being here for the first time without our tagalong is mitigated by the fact that the island feels so utterly altered. Cruz Bay is cleaned up but signs of the hurricane are everywhere: roofs torn off buildings, piles of rubble, smashed-up boats, trees ripped from their roots, favorite haunts blown apart, gone forever.

Every morning, Nick and I hike the Lind Point trail into Honeymoon Beach and have it all to ourselves for at least an hour. It's like being back in the 1990s, when we first started coming here, when we all fell in love with this place.

Nick takes pictures of island stonework as he works on his design for the mausoleum. He returns from a walk near the island cemetery one morning, enthusiastic about a tomb built in the classic St. John stone and brick style. He's taken a photo to show me.

I lean in to look. How have we come to be in such a place? Enthusiastic about a tomb. But "it's beautiful," I say. A bright blue glass heart inlaid into the stone. A young man who was also age thirty-three at his passing.

We decide to do our own quiet little "boat day," the first time it's ever been just the two of us, and I can't help but let my mind go to the boat day I had planned for that last trip with Caitlin and Andrew and Katie and Alvaro. We would have beelined over to Tortola to get through customs, then picked up some breakfast sandwiches in Soper's Hole, snorkeled at the Indians or the caves at Norman Island. Then conch fritters and rum punch at Pirates, on to Cooper Island for chicken rotis and more rum punch. A Sandy Cay swim, then over to the Soggy Dollar to wind up the day.

Now, little of that is possible anyway. From the boat, we get a clear view of the hurricane damage. The Caneel Bay resort looks like a place abandoned after an apocalypse. I take a photo of a room we'd once stayed in, its windows blown out, holes framing blue sky.

Over on Jost van Dyke, people are living in tents. On Great

Harbor's sandy main road, with the palm trees gone, everything looks too bright, too exposed. The church is destroyed, its roof and windows blown out. A tent with a pulpit and chairs has been erected beside it.

We end boat day, as we always have, on White Bay. A photograph of the Soggy Dollar Beach Bar was one of the first photos I saw posthurricane. STILL STANDING, they had posted.

The Soggy Dollar owners have already rebuilt the bar and planted new palm trees down along the beach. The sight is cheering, and we remember that Jess's sister's friend Annie is a manager at the Soggy Dollar. Her parents own the place. After Caitlin's service, Annie was the one who arranged an organ donor awareness day there, on New Year's Eve, in honor of Caitlin.

We ask if Annie's around. She is.

Annie is warm and kind. She hugs us and tells us that she lost her brother CJ six years ago.

Her parents live on St. John and we hope we will run into them, and St. John being such a small island . . . well, of course we run into her dad and other brother two days later. As talk progresses, we learn that the beautiful tomb that Nick admired and photographed is CJ's, the blue glass heart one of the favors at his island wedding.

And there is our newest synchronicity, and it feels like a blessing, happening as it has in our special family place. It really does.

In March, I receive an email from a friend of a friend, a science teacher who happens to be interested in mediums and in blind-testing them. She tells me about a book called *Surviving Death*, written by an investigative journalist.

This author brings up a variety of other paranormal events that are interesting, especially the reincarnation stories by Jim Tucker. I'll send you my favorite Jim Tucker video. He's a doctor at University of Virginia and has done some incredible research.

The medium readings that Katie, Shelley, and I experienced comforted me. All contained information no one could possibly know. Even so, my human brain hangs on to doubt.

I buy the book *Surviving Death: A Journalist Investigates Evidence for the Afterlife* by Leslie Kean. The author documents and provides thirty-plus pages of footnotes for her scrutiny of the UVA reincarnation investigations. The chapter about her experience with a medium also piques my interest. Kean ensured that her own reading was triple-blind anonymous and titled the chapter "An Almost Perfect Reading."

In all of our years in our home, we have rarely lost power because our house is on the police and fire grid in town. But as I am getting ready to leave for the writers' conference in Europe, we find ourselves deep into a nor'easter, the second one in a week, and for the first time in memory, we lose power. After twelve hours of no heat or electricity, we decide to spend the night in Caitlin's apartment in Boston, mainly because I'm concerned about Henry. He is fourteen and has always been healthy but now his vet is treating him for early kidney disease. He's been on a special diet and was doing well, but about two weeks ago, he stopped eating anything but the little bits of protein that were allowed in his food.

Once we arrive at Caitlin's apartment, Henry starts to deteriorate by the hour, so quickly that I am, at first, simply confused.

What is that funny smell? Why is he stumbling? At 2:00 a.m. he wakes me up, whimpering. He's had an accident.

I am numb. I know what's coming. I clean him and wrap him in the fleece blanket Caitlin used in the ICU. I sit in Caitlin's favorite spot on her sofa and hold him all through the night.

In the morning, we take him to the vet, and I've been afraid of this moment since the minute I first loved him. Miserable with grief, I kiss the top of his head and tell him, "You're going to see Caitlin now."

God, I hope that is true.

I have not always recognized happiness when I have had it in my hands, but sometimes my observing writer's brain prepares excruciating little gifts for my future self.

During my scrolls through my phone I find a video I took one day when I had some rare alone time in the apartment, Andrew and Caitlin gone off to a movie.

With the oxygen concentrator turned off, silence had transformed the space, made it hallowed. "These are the things you will one day miss," I'd said as the camera panned across the living room, the balcony, the kitchen, lingering over the blender that was in constant use, making those twice-a-day shakes, and there are the books that piled up, and the particular puzzle we were doing and her little leg-cycling unit, her two-pound weights, and the wooden Buddha she bought because she thought the all-white living room needed balance.

Henry's little food dishes. His kibble.

Everyday days, over forever.

At the writing conference in Positano, there will be three small workshops, with ten writers in each. I will be part of Dani's memoir group. Before I leave home, I receive the bound pages containing my group's work. They are in alphabetical order.

I begin to read the manuscripts, one per day. A few days before the conference, I am in London to visit Sinéad when I near the end of the manuscript. The Ws.

W. David Weill. The name seems familiar and I begin to read. And stop. I talk aloud to myself. "What? What is this? Are you kidding me?"

David is a pulmonologist and was the medical director of the lung transplant and adult cystic fibrosis programs at Stanford University for years. His manuscript consists of the first pages of a memoir he is writing about his complicated relationship with organ transplantation.

I also realize why I recognize his name. I text Mallory's mother in LA.

Is David Weill the Stanford lung doc friend you mentioned?

Yes, why?

And I tell her and she responds, *O my God, Mallory did an edit of his book.*

With the abrupt loss of Henry, my feeling of disconnection has intensified. But this coincidence is an affirmation, a powerful one. I am finding my path.

I'm not sure any other writing conference could be as magical as Sirenland, which takes place over a week at Le Sirenuse, a stunning Italian hotel that opens for the season every Easter, but soft opens for Sirenland before that, the owners being patrons of the arts who befriended Dani and her husband, Michael, a dozen years ago.

To get to Positano, a city pitched so vertically above the sea that to see it is a dizzying delight for the eyes, you follow a winding cliff road that hugs the Amalfi coast.

Once at Le Sirenuse, I stand on my balcony and take in the spectacular view I've seen in so many photographs. Now I am inside of it with a sense of expanding consciousness. Offshore are the Li Galli islands, where the Sirens sang to Odysseus as he sailed by, tied to his mast. Not far away are the ruins of Pompeii.

In Italy, I feel the smallness of my existence, the brevity and magic of a human lifetime, and it is a comfort.

After Italy, Nick joins me in England and we travel to more ancient places that Caitlin and I thought we would travel to after transplant: Salisbury Cathedral, Stonehenge, Bath.

The disbelief is still so strong that it almost feels like she's with us, and we end our week in London at a hotel where I twice stayed with Caitlin. I show Nick around the enchanting public spaces and point out areas that hold particularly vivid memories, such as the afternoon, in the lobby, when I realized that the man sitting beside me on the sofa was Cuba Gooding Jr. and he was sweet and funny and offered me a cake from his tiered tray, then shouted "BOO!" when I reached for one.

I show Nick where Caitlin got into the taxi with her big suitcase full of medical equipment that took her to the Chunnel train that brought her to Paris and the apartment where she spent those long-dreamed-of weeks alone.

After we unpack, we head down to the hotel's spa. Nick goes

to the men's changing area and I go to the women's. We arrange to meet on the thermal floor.

Once inside the changing area, the sights and spa smells are so immediately familiar. Caitlin is almost there, a shimmering memory in robe and slippers. I allow myself a moment, thinking, *The last time I was here, Caitlin was alive and* Cascade *was about to come out, and Cuba Gooding Jr. gave me a piece of cake. Life was pretty good.*

Then I go down to the thermal floor to look for Nick. It's kind of dark there and I don't see him, but suddenly he emerges through a door, followed by a man. "Look who I found!" he says, and it is Cuba, wrapping me in a hug, saying he is so sorry for the loss of Caitlin, and then he is gone, and my head is spinning a bit. Still is.

16

LITTLE MATCHES

No one ever told me that grief felt so like fear. Perhaps, more strictly, like suspense. Or like waiting; just hanging about, waiting for something to happen.

—C. S. Lewis, *A Grief Observed*

I have set a goal—a solid draft of this book by June 30—and the focus and immersion help. It connects me to Caitlin and disconnects me, a little, from the constant grief.

But then it happens. I am scrolling through my phone, looking for a photo, careful to avert my eyes when I know I'm near the photographs from those weeks in the ICU, but I miscalculate and land on something I am terrified to see: a picture of me, Nick, Andrew, Jess, and Penny, in yellow gowns and latex gloves and wearing masks, lined up beside Caitlin's bed. Caitlin unconscious in that frightening-looking way of those who've been unconscious for too long.

I had forgotten we had taken this photograph. December 18. The day of transplant. The last happy day.

I had said, "Let's take a picture. She will want a picture later."

A few swipes up and there she is in the same ICU bay, four weeks earlier during the time of the first offer, sitting up, holding Andy's hand, a nervous, hopeful smile on her face.

And it's too much. It's right back to the beginning, thrown-on-the-ground grief: she's gone, she can't come back, that waiting feeling I've been enduring, waiting for all this to be over, is false. I am never going to see her again.

*

This has been the week of suicides, of talk of suicides, of Kate Spade and Anthony Bourdain, and Facebook feeds with warnings and phone numbers, and I finally blurt it out to Nick, not teasing little bits the way I've been doing, but blubbering, wet-faced admission: I want to be dead. And if it were easy and not scary to do, I would gladly stop living. Because those stages of grief you read about, those guidelines—they have not fit with my experience. A year and a half later, the pain is as bad as it ever was.

Nick is kind. He cancels a few things. Hangs out with me. I tell him I've been meaning to call this trauma center I've heard about, and he urges me to do it.

He puts an arm around me and says, "Let's make the best of what we've got. There's plenty of time to be dead, bud."

*

In late June, I am sitting in a southern New Hampshire office park with Karissa the medium again. A few other people I know have now seen Karissa and we all feel comfortable with her. Today I just want to chat, ask the kinds of questions I've been able to ask Sinéad, such as "How do you do this? Do you hear? See?"

I sense that this is enjoyable for Karissa, too—to be able to talk about her work, as opposed to strictly doing it. She explains that although she hears *and* sees, she qualifies the seeing part. Seeing spirit isn't so much a lot of detail as it is the essence of the person, the soul, which is consistent across lifetimes, she says.

I tell her about Sinéad and about how Sinéad, since Caitlin passed, had been assuring me that I would *feel* her. I hadn't believed that, but now there's been some change. Recently, I say, I have sensed Caitlin when I've been in significant places and at the same time had a distinct and quite strong physical experience.

"It's this feeling like BubbleWrap," I say, "BubbleWrap that has been electrified. Like a grid, small squares."

When it started I was worried that something was wrong with my brain.

"Buzzing in my head. Super strong. It's always right here." I press my hand over the top left corner of my skull.

Karissa murmurs with understanding. She says that what I describe makes sense neurologically, that there's measurably more electrical activity happening in the mediumistic brain. "I've actually had a PET scan done on my brain while I was in a trance state and doing readings," she says.

When I ask for more information, she explains that she had it done by Dr. Jeff Tarrant, a psychologist board-certified in neurofeedback, who leads the NeuroMeditation Institute and authored *Meditation Interventions to Rewire the Brain: Integrating Neuroscience Strategies for ADHD, Anxiety, Depression & PTSD.*

"There's significantly more electrical activity happening in my brain, and in certain areas of the brain that are supposed to be shut off during waking states," she says. "There are two areas that are never supposed to be activated at the same time but in me they're both working while I'm 'reading.'"

She explains that she has a science background and that to have this bit of measurable data has been validating for her as well.

Her back is to the window. I am facing her, with a view to the outdoors, and as she talks, a hawk flies past the window.

A hawk. A white red-tailed hawk. I point. "Look!"

She smiles, but she is unfazed.

Later, I look up Jeff Tarrant and realize he is the doctor who Laura Lynne Jackson, a medium who has been blind-certified by the Forever Family Foundation and by the Windbridge Institute, wrote about in her autobiography. Laura devoted a section of her book to the brain scan she did with Dr. Tarrant. The brain mapping data results made sense to her, because they correlated with how she receives information in separate ways: psychically and mediumistically.

I am on a high after the conversation with Karissa. It released a lot of despair from the grief valve.

Over the next few days, I spend ecstatic hours on my phone watching videos that earlier would have had me sobbing. And as I look at Caitlin and listen to her, it's almost as if I'm with her.

That first summer of waiting, we'd sat in her Boston courtyard one night, trying to speak as if we had different accents—southern, French, Bostonian. In the videos, we laugh so hard, and I laugh so hard now, watching them. It feels good. Laughing feels good. I am normally a person who jokes and laughs a lot, and I haven't laughed in so long.

I clutch my phone, grateful for it. We live inside magic. We live inside a time in history when magic has become reality. I can look at that beloved face and hear that voice and think of the centuries of humans who had only memories after their loved ones died, and maybe a drawing or portrait or, more recently, photographs if they were lucky. I am reminded of a quote I read long ago, and which always stayed with me, by an English author named Eden Phillpotts, a man who was born in the 1860s: "The universe is full of magical things patiently waiting for our wits to grow sharper."

I end June unable to summon the despair I'd felt earlier in the month. I end June in a state of euphoria.

⬩

A few months ago, Nick ran across a call for artists for an annual juried outdoor art exhibition at a nature preserve in Southborough, Massachusetts.

Art on the Trails opens in late June.

Nick's installation is a grouping of three handcarved, heart-shaped boulders that lean against each other on a bed of stones. He's wrapped them in barbed wire, shot a big red hole straight through one of them, and cleaved another in half with a jagged red crack. *My Heart Hurts* will grace the entrance of the exhibit through late September. I ask him to write about it for the blog.

These past months, I smiled outwardly whenever family and friends approached or contacted me—I'm a lucky guy. Inwardly, I felt myself recoil more and more, as the hurt in my heart kept getting deeper and deeper.

Not sure why I entertained doing an art installation in Southborough, up the road from Fay School and St. Mark's, where Caitlin went to school.

I kept trying to make this a happy installation. At first I was thinking of something like a happy, smiling heart. But each day, working on this at our shop with my guys, I found myself in my office in tears.

I finally gave in as all the pain of these last 18 months came flooding in. The confusion, the names of friends dealing with their own hurting hearts. The hurt on Maryanne's face. The loss of Henry.

I finally realized that it is okay to say that my heart is hurting.

As painful as the construction process was, it was worth it that Wednesday at 2pm as I placed the final piece in place—a great relief and opening of my heart, I guess, as I smiled and thought, "Caitlin likes this" and I was so looking forward to Maryanne seeing it. As I walked away, two hawks soared above—Caitlin happy because her dad is.

⁕

Jess's breast cancer was aggressive enough that her oncological team has kept her on ongoing, oral chemotherapy. She encountered un-expected healing issues that have so far resulted in thirteen sur-geries. But with her team's okay, she has gone back to Kenya as often as possible, where she has been finding land and builders for a nonprofit she has established: The Leo Project in Honor of Caitlin O'Hara.

She plans to build an arts and resource center for vulnerable children, and asks me to look at some words she has written for the fund-raising page she is about to launch.

We were 31 and 32 when I was diagnosed with breast cancer. She knew more about medicine than most and she researched every-thing. I sent her all of my labs, my side effects, my questions. She was a well-curated vault of medical knowledge. She would have been an incredible doctor. I sent her screenshot after screenshot when a new drug was added to my regimen or I was deciding to taper off of something. She would talk me through each concern.

We talked about everything but when we were both sick, our conversations took on a new level of depth. We talked about death and about reincarnation; we talked about our purpose and spiri-tual inferiority.

On the evening of her 33rd birthday, we talked for hours and hours. I had just had another surgery and was tethered to my bed. She feared that her purpose here on this earth was to teach lessons to others.

"No. No," I said because I needed her here with me.

The idea that she was here only to teach others things was too much to bear.

I wonder if I would be as brave as Caitlin and Jess. I've had MRIs and panicked. I find small amounts of discomfort—a finger burn, nausea, sciatica—to be unbearable distractions that keep me so fo-cused on myself I can't think of anything else or remember what normal feels like. But I hope—and think—that we all are capable of finding sustained strength when necessary. Separating Caitlin and Jess and others with serious medical issues into a superhuman category makes it too easy for people to remember that pretty much everyone who has an issue was once someone who didn't.

An acquaintance of Nick's, same age, recently put his arm

around Nick one lovely spring day and said, *Oh, pal, I'm so sorry, I can't imagine* and then hours later climbed into bed and died.

I want to say to well-meaning people like that man, "Don't feel sorry for us. Just embrace what you have, right now, because you, too, are temporary."

Francis Weller is a psychotherapist who works with grief rituals and describes his clinical focus as soul-centered. He writes, "Every one of us must undertake an *apprenticeship* with sorrow. We must learn the art and craft of grief, discover the profound ways it ripens and deepens us."

I discover how much Caitlin was becoming practiced at this craft when I find, under a stack of books, a notebook she kept that last summer we were home, when she was fearing that her purpose on this Earth was to teach lessons to others. As usual with her, she'd only written on a few of the pages. The first one breaks my heart.

> *~I am so tired and freaked out. I am terrified.*
> *I want a sign.*
> *Anything. Answers. Give me something to give me faith.*

But the second page found her safe inside her brain, and I remember how much she meditated that summer. She listened to hypnotherapy apps and she seems to have recorded a rather mystical experience, a "conversation" of sorts with her uncle, Nick's brother Willie, the one who died when he was twenty-nine and left behind a one-year-old daughter, Meaghan.

> *~I want to ask Willie a question to see if he will answer.*
> *You have to come up with a question first.*
> *Okay. What was it like?*
> *It was hard and wet because it was raining.*

Can I ask another?
One more.
Last thing you thought of?
Meaghan.
One more?
A yes or no only.
Do you wish you could come back?
No.

On the third page, she had found some peaceful surrender.

~I feel like something relaxed in my brain. If we can/I can accept and see and know that it is all a construct, I can carry it all with me as one: the whole thing. There is no normal. No right way. No belief system. No one thing that works or doesn't, no answer. You know what is wrong and right, inherently. Follow that.

In July, we return to the Vineyard, to a different property, a former Methodist church and parsonage. The church, which is basically a very large bedroom now, is a sanctuary. Each morning I write at a long table and savor the fact that there is just the sound of wind in the trees, the calling of birds.

I begin a new practice with a notebook and instructions to myself that are rather simple: *Witness your response to each moment, and write down your observations, daily. Kindness to yourself is essential—no judgment.*

Of all the emotions I've felt these past months, anxiety has been the most difficult to fight. I've tried meditation, cannabis edibles, sound baths, deep breaths, measured breaths, wine.

Now the introspection helps. It's calming. Sometimes I write as if to Caitlin, and I listen for the practical, nonjudgmental wisdom that came so naturally to her.

One day toward the end of our time on-island, Nick and I are hiking through the woods to a pond. I say aloud, "I want to see an owl within the next twenty-four hours."

That night, we are reading in the church when I hear the distinctive whinnying trill of a screech owl. We've been here ten days and this is the first time I've heard an owl. I look up from my book, a big smile on my face. "Did you hear that?"

My sister and mother and nieces and many friends live in Maine, and whenever I am there, I arrange to see Andrew. In August we meet near Parson's Beach in Wells and I get in his pickup. We drive through Kennebunkport then park and sit on a bench near Walker Point, where we look out over the water and the town.

I've told him to never be afraid to tell me when he starts seeing someone, and now he tells me that he is seeing someone. He says she's very kind. And that it is good to have someone to talk to again, that he has felt very alone. And that he met her parents two weeks ago.

We are both a little choked up as he talks, and he puts his hand on my arm and I look at that kind, serious face. That face Caitlin loved. How I wish they'd been married. A son-in-law is so much more permanent than a boyfriend.

But I am happy for him and make that so known.

"This is all good, and as it should be," I say. Of course it is.

But when I get home, I cry and cry. I cry for two days.

Nick sends me a picture of three little kids. "Whose kids are these?" I ask, and he tells me but I'm looking at them and thinking, *More humans with bones and eyes. New humans.*

Do they spill and spill into the world for no reason? Or are there eternal souls behind those eyes?

Sometimes the years seem to sandwich together like glass slides in a science lab. You see all of them, clearly, one after another, so close you can almost live them, but that topmost layer of glass, that glass is the hard present.

Heading into the dread of a second anniversary, I put my head down and write this book; it's the only thing I can do, and when it overwhelms me, I tell myself, *One sentence at a time. Just keep at it.*

I am working on chapter 8, "An Unfinished Year," when in yet another synchronicity, Mallory's mother texts me to say that she's finished editing Mallory's memoir and that Penguin Random House will be publishing the book in March.

The subtitle of Mallory Smith's memoir, *Salt in My Soul*, is *An Unfinished Life.*

Nick and I have been spending the autumn binge-watching Masterpiece's *Poldark*. We've never watched so much TV here in our one-television home, but there's a lot of comfort in binge-watching, in giving ourselves over to make-believe.

Because I once looked up the show on my phone, I see a lot of *Poldark* in my so-called news feed. We are cooking dinner and I'm referring to a recipe on my phone when the newsfeed flashes a photo of Aidan Turner, the Irish actor who plays Poldark, waiting for a cab with his American girlfriend, Caitlin, thirty-five. If I squint, she could be our American Caitlin, age thirty-five now, living independently and gloriously. I look her up. This Caitlin grew up not far away, in Camden, Maine, and went to Concord Academy in Massachusetts. Both Caitlins probably have Independent School League friends in common.

I do this a lot lately: imagine the other lives we might have lived. The what-ifs. If our Caitlin had this other Caitlin's life, I wonder if I would have appreciated our good fortune. Oh, I probably would have given lip service to it, but I know that in my early days I was like most people: I believed that the truly bad things happened to others.

Even after the diagnosis, I told myself that Caitlin would be one of the fortunate exceptions to CF's rule.

Still, it was probably healthy to attempt to live happily and hopefully. We enjoyed a lot of good times.

I look up from my phone and watch Nick as he sautés the chopped mixture of clams and vegetables that is his specialty. I envision a spool of film extending out from the two of us, recording all the scenes of our life together. I think of our initial meeting in Ireland, how random it had seemed. I think of the other lives we might have lived, never knowing, never missing this one. And I think about soul groups, which Caitlin and I wondered about. The idea of soul groups feels right, makes sense. I'm feeling pretty sure that we were meant to meet, meant to be Caitlin's parents.

In the morning Nick says, "I went to sleep feeling very alone in the world."

"You're not," I say, "although we all are, in a way. But in the end, you're really not."

I've been wanting to get a close-up view of the first heart-lung machine, which I've been seeing through the window of Massachusetts General Hospital's medical museum whenever I pass by. I want another stark reminder that modern medicine is still pretty new. I want to feel lucky to have had Caitlin for as long as we did.

The heart-lung machine is gone, swapped out to make way for other exhibits. But I find myself transfixed by something suspended and otherworldly: a protein scaffold of a human heart, the possible future of organ transplantation.

A placard explains that this image, from the Ott Laboratory for Organ Engineering and Regeneration at MGH, depicts the process of "decellurization," which removes cells and leaves behind a protein scaffold. "This experimental process may be an alternative to traditional organ transplantation in the future. By using the donor organ's scaffold and seeding it with the recipient's own cells, the new organ could overcome the risk of the recipient's immune system rejecting a transplant."

A miracle, a dream. Science offering so much hope and yet deepening the mystery.

Yes, the mechanical function of the heart can be reproduced and genetic manipulation is advancing, but what of consciousness, emotion? The seat of the soul? Where is all that? The source of the pain of grief.

We are approaching two years. And two years is impossible.

⁂

The timeline of grief is not linear, and I'm learning that my openness about grief's persistence is valuable to others who are inclined to hide pain. But sharing is a balance, and I take care not to tip that balance over to my side. People ask how I am and I've taken to saying, in a normal voice, "It's just the hardest thing in the world, it's daily suffering. Thank you so much for asking. It's good to be able to share that."

Then—silence for a bit before, "And how are you doing?"

More often than not, the asker shares something important, too, and there we are: connected.

In the early days of our mourning, I had large postcards printed. They have a photograph of Caitlin on one side, space for writing and for an address and stamp on the other. Along the bottom, in black letters:

> *You think all this is important, but all that really matters is loving people and being kind.*

—CAITLIN ELIZABETH O'HARA, 1983–2016

I tell Nick that people who didn't know Caitlin are starting to romanticize that sentiment, as if it had come from a superhuman place of piety rather than from her tough core. He lifts an eyebrow and we both laugh. He says, "Then they didn't know that cat. She'd eat you for breakfast."

She would. And although I always felt proud of her fire, I think her character came entirely from within. Her life was wonderful, but it was never easy, and when what's important and what's not are made starkly clear, all the nonsense falls away. The point of life actually becomes simple, the truth of her simple admonishment profound.

We have oversize photos of Caitlin around the house, leaning up against various walls. We frequently look to them for moments of connection. "Good morning, Caitlin," Nick will say.

Most of the pictures are from preoxygen days, but a favorite is one that Andrew took in the fall of that last year in Pittsburgh. They were in Frick Park, a place they loved to visit because it had more than six hundred acres of hiking trails that were smooth enough that Andrew could push her in her wheelchair.

Caitlin laughed about those wheelchair trail rides. She said, "We must look *insane* out there, the wheelchair bouncing all over the place. Haha. Andy and Bad-Ass Kitten, hittin' the trails."

Bad-Ass Kitten. She liked to call herself that. In the photo, Bad-Ass Kitten is crouched next to a lean-to made of sticks, one hand on her oxygen tank, trees and trails behind her. She's smiling, wearing a head scarf and big white sunglasses. If not for the oxygen, you might think she'd built that lean-to, or at least planned to camp in it.

As always, making the best of her circumstances.

A good example.

December 16, 2012

CAITLIN: I think I need to go to New York
MARYANNE: Why
CAITLIN: To feel alive

On Christmas Day, Facebook reminds me that it cares about my memories! And here are some of them! Photos of our old bustling

Christmases, table set for fifteen or twenty, more coming later to the Barrel Party—crackling barrel full of fire, background of stars, moonlight, river ice, Irish coffee, laughter.

We wake up in New York City on this second Christmas, having decided to see what it's like to go somewhere and be alone. We drive home and eat the dinner our hotel boxed up for us. We watch a show on Netflix.

The next day Andrew is coming down from Maine for an overnight visit. At two o'clock that afternoon he texts me: *Leaving Maine now.*

I am alone in the house and I let myself imagine that he is with Caitlin, that she's phoning from the car and I speak my side of the conversation, aloud.

Hi bud. I can't wait to see you!

Coquille St. Jacques. Irish potatoes. Daddy's making those. And oh, I don't know, what would you like, broccoli?

Okay. Okay!

I love you.

Please drive safely.

I imagine hanging up and then double over with the pain I've inflicted on myself.

I have always had a good imagination. I imagined that conversation so well that a little while later I experience a moment of confusion. What if it was true? What if I've been inside a nightmare and Caitlin's really on her way home? What is this terrifying uncertainty?

Nick arrives home as I stand at the stove, stirring crème fraîche into a mirepoix I am preparing for the scallops. He asks how I am.

I double over again. "I'm having a hard time," I say.

17

FAITH IS A CHOICE

12/31/2018

MARYANNE: Where are you?

Early in the new year, my brother comes by for Sunday dinner. He mentions he recently found a little drawing he'd done of me in 2014, when Caitlin was first so sick.

"I felt so bad for you," he says. "You had this look on your face, and I pictured you backed up against a ledge, in armor and with wings."

I ask him why he hadn't shown it to me back then.

"You always complain that I draw you with a big nose."

I laugh. "Please send it," I say. I want this visual proof of what I suppose I really do know: that we are all stronger than we realize.

"I'll see if I can find it."

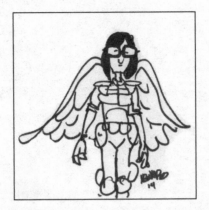

MICHAEL: I described the drawing being more spectacular but I guess that's how I felt when I drew it. I found it in a pile of drawings and doodles.

MARYANNE: I like that you did it and what it represents.

MICHAEL: It was right after I visited you and didn't know how to express myself.

MARYANNE: Well you did.

MICHAEL: ♥

1/7/2019

MARYANNE: I just booked tickets to LA. It will be good to see Mallory's parents.

KATIE: So much in common. Two beautiful, sharp girls. UPMC. Transplant.

KATIE: The strongest thing in my eyes has been the willingness to share.
To willfully immerse yourself over and over in the memories.
To struggle with making sense and meaning not just intimately, interiorly, but in public. In the book. For other people.
KATIE: How have you mothers survived this!?

⁂

While we waited for transplant, I wrote a novel. One of the characters in it—a woman that I lived with for three years and then abandoned in December 2016—was an oral historian in Washington, DC. She has been rapping on my head these past weeks, so I open "Camera-Eye.doc" and look for her. In the scene I've been thinking about, she is telling David, a kind of lost soul, that oral histories are important, that people need to tell their stories, need to have those stories heard, and that humans need purpose in their lives. I find the page and read the words: "If you were suddenly completely alone on Earth, would you want to live? You could be surrounded by all the things that people had made—paintings and poems and musical recordings and film and it would all be lovely and unbearable."

Most people in our life understand that as Caitlin's existence recedes ever further into the past and we are forced into the future, grief persists. The younger people—Katie and Jess and Caitlin's cousins Sinéad and Jillian and Melissa—are particularly conscious of this. As are her friends. Alyssa invites us to a dinner party. Kate Ryan prints her correspondence with Caitlin and has it bound in a beautiful book. Elizabeth sends the kinds of cheerful cards she used to send to Caitlin in Pittsburgh. Billy writes rambling, wonderful, middle-of-the-night emails. Alex sends flowers on Mother's

Day. Mieke says, "Let's get a date on the calendar for you to come upstate." Kenley pops over every time she's home from Brooklyn.

In her Mother's Day post in 2015, Caitlin had written, "When you get evaluated for transplant, part of the evaluation is making sure you have a good support system, because it is so vital to how well you do. This might seem hard to grasp to a healthy person who thinks that ultimately, you can get through anything on your own if you really have to. I am telling you—haha—you can't. You need people."

I'm here to tell you it's true. You survive because people help you survive.

❦

I don't want to die, although I am now more curious about it. I think, *One day I will know! Or not . . .*

Katie and I laugh about that. "I don't want to die, of course I'm not ready to die," she said one night. "But now I'm kind of excited to see what happens."

If consciousness continues, I imagine it thus: an emerging, an awareness, a lifting of amnesia. Great relief. *Thank God that's over!*

If it doesn't, I imagine a soft stop, a blurred-edges ache of an end, like the closing paragraph of F. Scott Fitzgerald's *Benjamin Button* story.

The thought of eternal life used to horrify me. Instinctively, from my earliest considerations of the idea, I thought, *No! Wrong!*

But existence on another plane, a soul life, as opposed to this hard human life—that's palatable. Worth contemplating.

❦

In California, the thirty-threes and other signs are so nonstop I don't know what to make of them.

If before they were like fireflies on a summer's night, now they are the Perseid meteor shower. On our first day, I am walking down Abbott Kinney Boulevard in Venice, California, leaving some impromptu voice messages for Sinéad. Now that the book is nearly finished, I say, I want to think about the healing garden, and what about a small, travelers-wagon-type caravan? Fitted out with trays for plants and flowers? As I am speaking, just such a caravan pulls up and parks. It is small and round and looks Tolkienesque, with tiny paned windows and hanging lanterns. It has a name: Tin Can Tarot.

I stare at it a moment. I'm stupefied, and at the same time, my mind is working. I imagine it full of plants. Dirt. Organisms. Not good for sick people to breathe. Then I meet Nick for lunch, where the maître d' tells the hostess, "Put them at table thirty-three," and the day's printed menus are illustrated with a drawing of a cat.

After our meal I go back to Tin Can Tarot for a reading. I ask a general question about my book project. I draw the seven of pentacles, the three of swords, the chariot, the ace of cups, the lovers—cards that say I've sown the seeds, done the work, and after some initial disappointment I must take focused action and stick to my own vision of the book, and if I do, the project will go very well, and that spreading the message in my book will be almost like a calling for me.

Okay.

A calling. And what is this calling to be? The answer comes, one I've heard before. *You're supposed to help people into the next life.*

Back on the sidewalk, I pause next to a shop to text Nick. When I look up from my phone, my eyes meet David Bowie's, looking out at me from the cover of a biography that sits on a chair behind the shop's spare display window. Lying in front of the book is a black T-shirt imprinted with one word: "BREATHE."

Inside, the shop is as spare as its window, offering an eclectic mix of goods: a couple of books, a few items of clothing, a smattering of home goods. There is one other biography for sale, its subject Leonard Cohen. And one other T-shirt, this one printed with the tarot card I've just held in my hand: the ace of cups, a card that depicts a flat palm holding a chalice overflowing with abundant water.

Moments later, a customer begins spelling her name to a store clerk: "C.a.i.t.l.i.n. . . ."

"You're not going to believe all this," I say to Nick when we meet up. "Look," he says, and points at the car parked in front of us, the "3333" on its license plate.

Days of synchronicities follow: noir photographs of Joni Mitchell that greet us when we arrive at the Hotel Bel-Air for a drink. Hawks. Owls. Bolting awake at 3:33 a.m. with the answer to a book problem that has been eluding me. Meeting Christina, a writer friend, for tea, and realizing that her editor is the same editor who is publishing Mallory Smith's book.

It's as if the signs are batting at me: *Hey you, don't you remember? Don't you remember the knowing you had as a child? Remember "Have faith"?*

<hr />

We travel to Santa Barbara, a town so beautiful, with its cream-colored buildings and orange mission-tiled roofs, its towering palms by the bay, that you realize why so many people migrate to this state.

Late in the evening we are reading when we remember that there's a total lunar eclipse happening tonight, a super blood moon.

Our room is on the top, fourth floor of our hotel. Across the hall, double doors lead to a balcony with benches and cushions. A young couple is out there watching. As we step outside, I grab Nick's arm with astonishment. "O my God! I've never seen such a moon!"

The couple glance back and smile. *Right?*

The moon hangs close and red in the sky, like something supernatural, so near we can see its topography. My eyes soak it in and it's like being a child again, looking at the world and shivering with delight, thinking, *What is all this wonderful beauty?* When I finally look away, I see that all along the streets below us, people have stopped to look, too, heads tilted back like humans have done since humans existed.

We are all connected, safe inside eternity.

5/12/2016

Caitlin: *In reading* Sarum *it makes reference to this house in the 1400s being built on the same site as the house that Porteus had built 1000 years ago (and about 250 pages ago). It seems so crazy to me that me and this 1400s man are more closely related in time than he and Porteus. I love thinking about stuff like that.*

In my hotel room I open my computer and read through the transcript of my session with Karissa. I make a list of the direct messages and contemplate each one.

* My poor mom, she's waiting to have this "experience" with me. Trust me. It's coming, not in the way you think it is, it's never going to be on your timeline.

* What's it going to take for you to feel like this is real?
* This is the new dawn of you learning to live with me in a different way.
* Grief is the most deafening sense of loneliness that can come over anybody.
* Listen to Joni Mitchell. Let me speak to you in Joni.
* You have to pick up on the self-care again. And I'm watching you.
* I am the hawks.
* Faith is a choice.

Maybe surrender is the answer, the way to make the rest of life not only bearable, but also good.

Meditating is a kind of surrendering, and meditating these past months has helped. The easeful mind-set stays with me in such a way that in a rough moment, I can slow down, breathe a conscious breath, blank my mind, reflect.

What I now reflect on is this idea that faith is a choice. I've never considered faith to be the kind of thing one chooses, but the more I consider it, the more I see that faith, that great paradox, can *only* be a choice.

Long ago, after Caitlin was diagnosed with CF, I decided that I wouldn't "ruin today worrying about tomorrow." Most of what we worry about generally doesn't happen, and even when it does, worrying never helps.

Similarly, I can "choose faith." If I tune out the human world with its noise and skeptics and focus on my gut, I find moments of deep, internal *knowing*. I can imagine her with me always, live as though her soul endures. Otherwise I might live out the rest of my days in terrible sorrow, grieving that I will never see her again, and then, when my time to cross over comes, see how wrong I was.

I might instead live with gratitude for what I did have. Live purposefully. Start to "help people into the next life" by sharing this decision to choose faith. I can share the signs—people take comfort in them. I can train for the hospice volunteering I've long been drawn to do.

And the big share is that I have so much of Caitlin's wise mind at hand. I can hold up her glowing example of how to live, how to be. I'm still receiving messages from strangers who thank me for writing about her, and from Caitlin's friends who say they often ask themselves, what would Caitlin do, say? Caitlin helps them live their lives more bravely, and with better intention.

I read over the vast tapestry of her ruminations, texts, emails, and notes, and see a constant, thick, bright thread: Caitlin was always striving for goodness.

Goodness. A word that is like a North Star.

From: Caitlin
To: A friend with a strong religious faith
Date: May 18, 2014
Subject: Faith

Can I ask you something personal? If you don't want to answer I understand. I have never been that religious but I have always had faith. I hope that makes sense to you. As I get older I struggle more and more with the reality side of my brain and the side that wants to hope and pray for the best, and have faith. I am always so interested in how people like you—really smart people, that is—stay so solid in their beliefs and faith. I don't know, I guess I am just curious about it. Sometimes things happen that make me feel like I am more connected and that it is possible. I've been trying this thing where I "dialogue" with my illness. It was recommended by an astrologer who did my chart, and it is something I kind of do a lot anyway but in a different way. It's like visualizing sessions of going through your body and imagining healing. But this takes it a step further with actual talking to your disease. Anyway I was lying in bed this morning doing that for like half an hour. Andrew was there, he was like half awake, we were just laying around. Anyway I never said I was doing that. Then when he got up and was walking into the living room he just said casually, "I feel like God was in the room this morning." It was so odd, that is not a normal thing for him to say (obviously). It was just kind of cool.

I am pretty open about everything, but religion is one thing where I am both curious and less knowledgeable. There is so much craziness around religion, that I am always compelled by the smart and grounded ones who find their faith in it, like you. And there have certainly been times when I have reached for it (and it is Christianity, because that's what I was raised with, however weakly).

When I got older I got interested in reincarnation. Stories of children remembering details of lives that they couldn't possibly have known, the idea that we are here to learn lessons in this life. Figure out what those lessons are, be good people, and evolve our souls. The idea of souls. It was fun to read about, yes, but mostly the ideas of reincarnation resonated with me. I was interested in the fact that most of the religions embraced the idea very early on in their inception (or so I have read), and even though now it is considered maybe "new age-y" it was in fact very "old age-y."

When I was very sick that time, my mother had an experience

of lying on the couch in our living room sobbing, just crying really hard. Thinking, how will this ever be ok. She said she heard a voice say clear as a bell "have faith." She has told me this story lots of times since then. She says it was so clear she sat up immediately and stopped crying. Yesterday she bought me a card. She picked it based on the quote on the cover by Frances Hodgson Burnett (author of the Secret Garden) "Hang in there. It is astonishing how short a time it can take for very wonderful things to happen." She came home and opened it to give it to me and inside it said "Have Faith." She didn't even know that . . . how odd?! And wonderful.

Anyway—things like this, and the moment with Andrew, are just examples of many validating moments I have had during whatever my spiritual journey is. They have made me believe that there is something there. Sometimes I am more connected to it, and sometimes I am not. Perhaps that is the drawback of not having a solid religion to keep you connected, to draw from when you feel like you are losing faith. I don't know. This might all sound insane to you. I don't want to think of myself as one of those people that everyone seems to be nowadays which is just "I'm spiritual but not religious," because I think it is more than that. It is more than just liking the idea of something. I think you have to believe in the GOOD of something, solidly, in order to stay the course.

So. Faith is a choice, and life is either random and often quite cruel or there is more to life than this life and somehow, in a way that no one can explain or disprove, consciousness endures and meaning is a real thing. That we come to this life with some kind of rough map, with familiar guideposts along the way and wiggle room to make choices.

Life itself is so magical that it's not that much of a stretch to believe that there is at least one other level higher than this particular reality of a life span on Earth.

If we consider the premise that our souls chose these lives, planned these courses of lessons, if that is true, then we can figure out the challenges we might have set for ourselves. We can see those challenges and lessons with great clarity. Our reaction to adversity softens, becomes more accepting. And every moment of living can have purpose, meaning.

<hr />

A book has to end, even if grief doesn't know that.

There's no big conclusion here, but as I write these final pages, the little signs are all around me. Thirty-threes everywhere. A hawk that lands on our patio table and looks at Nick. A ringtone playing the old Meow Mix jingle so loudly through speakers that our incredulous attention is called to the name of the boat behind us in the St. John harbor that Nick and I are in: *Nine Lives*, the name of my blog. I am talking to my agent about this book and an instrumental "Hallelujah" begins to play on the sound system, so quietly I think I must be imagining it. I click on a *Boston Globe* article about hospice volunteers and realize, *That's it—that's where my portable healing garden might fit in*. I don't have a chance to read the story for a few days, and when I finally get to it on this bright Saturday morning, it has accrued thirty-three comments and a line jumps out at me: "Brother Paul O'Keefe's mother spent 15 years toward the end of her life ministering to people on hospice who were afraid to die. She offered friendship. They had questions about God. She sat with them even if she had no answers."

Little matches, lighting up the dark.

Caitlin liked to pull back and picture herself and our planet in time and space. She wrote, "It makes me removed enough to ultimately feel that there is not much I can do to change the shifts of the world, but also inspired enough to think—what is my role in this lifetime?"

Now it's my turn.

If these lifetimes are for growing the soul, there's work to be done.

AFTERWORD

For those who would like a bit more: pieces by or about Caitlin.

❧

Caitlin's Laptop, Open Windows

what on earth could i have to say?
how much should we self reflect?

wild rice

quinoa

papaya

Redemption Song

what kind of country are we? I want to be my own nation"—a character in Homegoing says. My mind can't make sense of killing to protect a nation. It's not my mind actually. It's something else. My soul? My mind can understand it. We live in a nation and we want the protection and rights it affords us so we have to be willing to fight for that. People want to harm us. . . . I would want to fight for freedom. It's not anti fighting. But as a person, deep down, can you ever really reconcile that? Or is that all part of being human? Having to live with the reality that your life might mean someone else's death. In any scenario.

❧

Note Found Among Caitlin's Papers

LITTLE BIRD DRAWING BY CAITLIN, 2014

June 26, 2016

When I hear music, I fear no danger. I am invulnerable. I see no foe. I am related to the earliest times, and to the latest.

—H. D. THOREAU

I love this, because it captures that something that has always brought me comfort of being able to feel like I was connecting with it all—to the people who came before, and lived it, and endured it, survived, but eventually died. It's all so commonplace what we go through. It takes the weight out of it, the darkness, but also adds an overwhelming poignancy and urgency to now. Tight string from then to now. So easily broken, but when you pluck it, it makes music—like moments of life.

❦

On Nature

To: John B. Mulliken, MD, FACS, FRCS, Eng (Hon.)
From: Caitlin O'Hara
August 13, 2015

Dr. Mulliken,
I am the person from the Prouty group to whom you sent your generous donation for the Prouty Garden. Again—*thank you.*

We are adding the offline donations made to our current tally on our fundraising site—it is simply so that our fundraising amount to date will accurately reflect the money we have received, from all avenues. When listing your donation, would you prefer that I list it as anonymous? Or do I have permission to use your name? Either is fine.

Thank you again—your words at the Gathering made me stand up out of my seat when I watched them, and want to proclaim YES! —my uncle was the guy behind the camera :) It is so encouraging to see physicians come forward and speak up for the Prouty. I'm a 30 year CF patient at Children's, and though the idea of "thinking outside the box" is more commonplace now, back when I was much younger, my beloved Dr. Wohl taught me to always be thoughtful, and to never fall back on a preconceived certainty. I watched her do it with all her decisions with me, thinking seriously, and often admitting when she wanted to change course—this after 40 years of practice. I also saw her aggressive medicine save my life at one point, and at the same time, it was the Prouty that inspired me to get up and walk, days after surgery, carrying chest tube boxes. Both were integral to my and my parents' ability to stay sane, have hope, and draw goodness from our experience then, and throughout my life with CF, and I know both have been a part of my making it this far. I so so appreciate when physicians really understand that. I have tried to be thoughtful throughout my involvement in trying to save the Garden—and ask myself continually, is it the right thing? I keep finding my answer is yes.

I am waiting now for a lung transplant at UPMC, and though it's going to be this wild miracle of science, and surgeons, that make me healthy, it is *nature*, here in Pittsburgh (the Frick gardens, Frick park, Lake Erie), that has kept me going, mentally and subsequently physically, for these past 15 months of waiting. It will be those things that help get me through my recovery. There are no patient gardens at UPMC (there is one, brick, pocket roof patio near a vent), and when I am inpatient it is very difficult—it makes me work even harder for the Prouty.

Forgive me for going into so much detail, but as a patient, I wanted you to know how much I appreciated your presence at the gathering, not just your donation.

Best,

Caitlin

A Matter of Ethics

Draft of the letter intended for the Brigham and Women's Hospital lung transplant team, 2016

I grew up outside Boston, and have been a patient at Children's since I was diagnosed at age 2 with CF, in 1985. Once an adult, I transitioned to inpatient treatment at Brigham and Women's Hospital (BWH).

In spring of 2006 I was still "too healthy" for transplant, but I began the process at BWH at my doctor's urging. BWH was one of the hospitals who transplanted cenocepacia patients like me—along with UPMC, Cleveland Clinic, Duke, and a handful of others. "Better to get started early" was the thinking, "so that when you get really sick, you are ready to be listed." I began the evaluation as an outpatient and completed a significant amount of its required tests. I continued to remain fairly stable in my health.

Then, in 2008, an administrative assistant from BWH called me, out of the blue, as I was getting ready for work, and told me they would no longer be able to offer me a spot for transplant because of my cenocepacia. Things spun for a minute—"No," I argued. "You already know I have cenocepacia, we've been over this, your program takes cepacia patients."

There had been a change in policy, the woman said.

I wasn't sure what to think. I was confused before I could be upset. The woman said I should have received a letter. I hadn't, although it did arrive in the mail, weeks later—simple and boilerplate—another baffling link in the chain of events. Soon, almost all of the other hospitals began to deny transplant to cenocepacia patients. I grew panicky.

Eventually, I worsened and did my evaluation at UPMC. I was listed on April 24, 2014. Because I would need to reach UPMC in four hours, we set up emergency jet service (which is never a guarantee), and began to wait. When December came, my mother and I moved to Pittsburgh to "wait out the winter."

Winter passed. May of 2015 found me sick and in the hospital. It made no sense to go home at that point, and surely I would be called soon, was the thinking. We reluctantly signed a new lease on an apartment.

A year passed.

I have now been listed at UPMC for 2 ½ years. It's taken an incredible emotional and financial toll on my family. I own an apartment in Boston, right around the corner from the hospital, that sits empty while I wait here.

So why did all of this suddenly happen?

A study in the American Journal of Transplantation in 2008 concluded this:

> Cooperation between CF treatment and LT centers will hopefully provide new insights into virulence, transmissibility and treatment regimens for this unique and challenging pathogen. More specifically, further studies to identify which specific strains of B. cenocepacia may be more virulent, the mechanisms behind the virulence in such strains and investigations to tease out what host factors might influence progression of the infection in the CF population should be a priority. Until then, we recommend the careful screening of all CF patients for BCC and excluding from LT those harboring B. cenocepacia, regardless of susceptibility profile.

That conclusion, and recommendation, was made **despite** the fact that the study was based on a very small group of people with cenocepacia—7. Of those 7, 3 died of Burkholderia-related complications, 2 died of other transplant complications, and 2 were . . . alive. The data of these 7 individuals was taken from groupings of people who were transplanted between 1992–2002, a time span that began 16 years prior, when many programs were just beginning to offer transplants, and ended 6 years prior to the study's date of publication. The group of non-burkholderia CF patients used as comparison was a study of 59 patients. 9 cultured other forms of BCC, and as mentioned before, 7 harbored cenocepacia.

Being that there are so few studies on cenocepacia and their outcomes, and even fewer at the time the article was written in 2008, the conclusions drawn cast a wide net across the transplant community. I personally was immediately removed from the transplant evaluation at Brigham and Women's. I was upset, but it would still be a couple of years before the reverberations of this decision were truly felt, when I got much sicker. For some, they were already being felt, and for others they meant the arrow pointing towards death was now certain.

This situation is a serious matter of ethics.

The blanket exclusion of one very small group of people from almost all centers, based solely on the organism that they culture, is ethically wrong. Not only is the data presented about cenocepacia and transplant anecdotal and outdated, but the process of eliminating one very small minority group like this on that outdated evidence is directly in contrast with the typical "case-by-case basis" methodology of evaluating patients at most centers.

Transplant centers certainly must reserve the right to evaluate and accept, or reject, transplant candidates. **But it should be on a case by case basis.**

Where is the logic in being pointed in the direction of certain death, because the risk of possible death is too great in the other direction? Is that what lies at the core of medicine? Balancing risk, but to a fault?

To those who say "it's a complicated issue," I say, "It's not, it's a simple issue, with a complicated story." At 33, I have end-stage CF that ends with certain, early death. There exists a potentially life-saving surgery available, but because this surgery includes a risk of death, I am being denied opportunity for it by nearly every center in the country. When a man is drowning, does the man on shore say "I can't save you, we could both drown?" Sometimes he does and he has to live with himself, because that person will certainly drown without help. This is even simpler than that. No surgeon will die if I die, no doctor or caregiver. Is my chance at a year, or two, or five at life, worth less than someone else's? Who gets to "decide" who uses organs "to the fullest"? I challenge you to ask anyone who has had a transplant if they'd do it all over again even if they knew they would die after only a year, and you will hear a resounding, unanimous, YES.

UPMC Pittsburgh practices real medicine. This transplant team is not in the business of cherry-picking the candidates they deem most likely to survive, in order to improve their statistics. Instead, they accept high-risk, last-resort patients like me, in an attempt to save our lives. I am grateful to my team: my compassionate pulmonologist, Joseph Pilewski, and the brilliant surgeons, Drs. D'Cunha, Shigemura, and Hayanga.

Caitlin

The Hardware Store Cat, a Story
By Caitlin, October 2016

Mr. Humphreys wheezed along the hot sidewalk of his new West 81st street neighborhood, then headed into the hardware store where, much to his asthmatic dismay, the resident Persian sat.

Humphreys, with a measured inhale, made an attempt to enjoy the blast of air-conditioned cool while at the same time filter out what he imagined as "cat air"—air that seems pure but in truth is littered with bits of catty flecks that would set off a chain of respiratory events.

The cat, named Frosty according to her bowl, appearing

to sense Humphreys' distress, rose to leave—but was frozen, stuck to the stool. For what Humphreys did not know—nor did the cat until this very moment!—was that Frosty had been sitting on that stool for 15 years.

Why, only now, had Frosty become so corporeally aware? She was anxious as Humphreys came to her, holding his breath but revealing love in his eyes as he wrested her, with large and dusty hands, from her sclerotic position.

Humphreys' move had been automatic. He shook out of the trance and braced himself as he let go of his breath and mentally braced for the deep inhalation of concentrated cat air that was sure to follow. But he breathed in and nothing happened—nothing at all. . . . For in those 15 years Frosty had become special, free of irritants and organic matter, like a living sphinx—the kind of rare cat that finds only those who can truly love her—the asthmatics and the allergics of the world who have long pined for a cat they cannot love with heart nor lung. For them, there is the hardware store cat.

* * *

Thoughts on the Night

From: Andrew
To: Maryanne
Date: 1/20/2017
Subject: The night

I think a lot about the time Caitlin spent only with herself, usually between midnight and 8am. I may have been present but predictably in a deep slumber.

I know this time involved a lot of suffering. She couldn't sleep unless she was propped up by 6 or 7 perfectly stacked pillows. The trips to the bathroom to pee were slow and frequent. When she did sleep, it was regularly haunted by nightmares. She would sometimes wake up suddenly in a fit of coughing, unable to get back to sleep. She had a lot of tricks her little body taught her to mitigate these bed time miseries.

It sounds awful, and it was. But if you asked Caitlin what her favorite part of the day was, she would tell you it's the night. She loved the alone time, it was all hers.

Caitlin's Service Program

Caitlin Elizabeth O'Hara
Born Sunday, July 31, 1983, in Framingham, MA, 1:17 a.m.
Leo Sun, Aries Moon, Gemini Rising

Soul departed on Tuesday, December 20,
2016, 6:28 p.m., in Pittsburgh, PA

Early Christian art, northern Renaissance art, all art, Henry, Joni Mitchell, all music, classical piano, good movies, the work of Martin Scorsese, good television, the brilliance that was *Mad Men*, good books, philosophy, birds—all birds, even pigeons, especially pigeons, Audubon's work, Paris, the city of light. Nights at Sorrelina with Mummy. St. John. Home. The smell of JP Licks. The smells of the beach and barbecue and bourbon. Menemsha, steamers at Larsen's, the Ag Fair, Buddy the Elf what's your favorite color?, Henry, pup jokes, pups, movie line jokes, "whish wigs?," *Groundhog Day*, "I'm NOT goin' back to Pittsburgh," Shopbop, astrology, being Leo, three little pigs, pig room, pig chairs, soft sweaters, LLBean slippers, head scarves, cats, all animals—the more sad and forlorn, the better—donkeys on St. John, boat days on St. John, drives out to the East End, Ivan's, Soggy Dollar, the *Gilligan's Island* cay, Seabreeze. Ireland. Barn owls, all owls. Daddy days. The Fort. Lucy and Rickey tap tap tap and Laura 6:00 a.m. Sleeping in. Staying up late. Going to the cinema, Roger Ebert, onion rings, comfort, warm socks, foot massages, leg massages. Being in charge/the boss. Making lists. Reiki, "We're connected." 7A sausage breakfast sandwiches, llamas, Miami, the Standard, day trips, Kennebunkport, Girls, the green couch, Simba, Talking Heads, Judy. Buying gifts for friends. Writing beautiful, handwritten notes. The ocean. Salt. Peace. Equality. Fairness. Feminism. Underdogs! Chugging water. Raggedy loungewear. Rags. Dancing. Singing—singing out loud. Popcorn. Butter. Berries. Baby chicks. Kindness. Crying. Chatting. Take-out. High-end stuff. Gypsies. Babies. The unknown. Religion. Spirituality. Boston. The Vineyard. Cats. Bob Dylan. Bobby McGee. Brownies. Books. Small creatures. Love. Travel to old Europe, the churches—the older and more ornate, the better. Genealogy, pearl earrings, corndogs at the fair, Henry, the Newton cemetery, Mary Oliver, Easter candy, pig pups, rabbit rabbit, the Virgin Mary, watermelon sherbet, snails, spirit animals, the small white flowers that smelled so wonderful at the UPMC hospital garden and which were the smell of childhood, parrot tulips, the good articles in *The New*

Yorker, pies, driving around listening to music, Prouty Garden, DonandKay all one word, Toulouse, Berthe, Lake Champlain chocolate caramel bars from Whole Foods, Chinese food delivery, Henry, dozens of wrist bracelets, being alone to sit and think, driving to Castle Island to look at the harbor, road trips, Maine, the first year with Andrew in the Ogunquit apartment. Andrew.

Only humans can understand goodness and beauty in a way that can change us.

—CAITLIN

ACKNOWLEDGMENTS

Oh, so many to thank and not enough ink to pen my gratitude to every person, loved ones and strangers alike, who supported us. Firstly, my gratitude to Caitlin's years of medical teams at Boston Children's Hospital, Brigham and Women's Hospital, and the University of Pittsburgh Medical Center. In particular, Craig Lillehei, the late Mary Ellen Wohl, Ahmet Uluer, Joseph Pilewski, Erin Pulcini, Samantha Thompson, Lara Schaheen, Penny Sappington, and Jonathan D'Cunha. And, of course, Laura Kelly.

Thank you to my sister, the faithful Kate, and all of my extensive family, to Diane and my many precious friends, and to all of Caitlin's beloveds. Each of you provided connection, support, love, and ferocious positivity when we needed it most.

I do not even know the names of all of the people who were involved in the chain of goodness that coordinated pleas throughout the land during those desperate days that we searched for lungs, but please know this: I love every one of you.

To every kind stranger who has continued to connect with us, in creative and thoughtful ways—thank you.

Thank you for permission to use correspondence or portions of personal stories: Andrew Sutryn, Jess Danforth, Katie Whittemore, Kate Ryan Baird, Renu Linberg, Meg Heneberry, Heather Hunter, Amanda St. Lawrence, Kate Schell, Patrick Connelly, Beecher Grogan, John Mulliken, Larry Boggs, Teppany Skinner-Aguillera and Kwesi Aguillera, Shelley Senai, Kat David, Carole DeSanti, Rachel Priselac, Elizabeth Kemper French, Sylvia True, Sirrý Berndsen, Karissa Dorman, and the family of Hillary Stanton Foulkes.

To the Friends of the Prouty Garden and its thousands of supporters, and especially "Uncle Mike"—you helped give purpose to Caitlin's last years. The good karma you spread during that time will be with you always.

Thank you to Susan Conley for true friendship and for reading my pages every Monday, to soul buddies Jane McCafferty and Monique Hamze for steady encouragement, to Sinéad de hÓra for being my earth angel, and to Shelley Senai and Katie Whittemore for laboring over the particulars with me.

Thank you to the O'Hara and Company crew—Linda and all the "men at work"—and to all of Nick's colleagues in the Boston design and construction world who made life easier for us.

Thank you to the team at HarperOne who turned my manuscript into the beautiful book I envisioned, and to Stephanie Cabot, who knew that Mickey Maudlin would be the perfect editor for *Little Matches*. He was. Thank you, Mickey. Thank you, Stephanie. My special thanks also to Chantal Tom, Ellen Goodson Coughtrey, and to Nicole Dewey. I am grateful that fate led me to Dani Shapiro's intelligent and soulful writing retreats—the magic atmosphere she conjures was part of the genesis of this book.

Shane Volney, thank you for providing us with the iconic, light-filled photograph of our Kitten. And Winky Lewis, thanks for taking the perfect photograph of my endpapers tableau.

I will always be in awe of how *good* are the people of Pittsburgh, and want to offer special thanks to Ralph and Mary Cindrich and all the Cindriches, to all our kind neighbors at 151 Fort Pitt Boulevard, and to Jane McCafferty, Jane Bernstein, Maggie Jones, Jim Stanley, Joni Kamen, and Ken and Sara Segel and the Squirrel Hill Jewish community.

Thank you to Nick for being a solid, loving, and honorable dad and husband, and for being the kind of person who "builds it beautiful, builds it to last."

And finally, to those who grieve Caitlin's donor, my enduring condolences and my deepest thanks.

FURTHER READING

Here is a list of some of the books and resources that I refer to in the book.

Contemplative Nonfiction

Bauby, Jean-Dominique. *The Diving Bell and the Butterfly* (New York: Vintage, 1996).

Emerson, Ralph Waldo. "Self-Reliance," essay in *The Portable Emerson* (New York: Penguin Books, 2014).

Frankl, Viktor E. *Man's Search for Meaning* (Boston: Beacon Press, 2006).

Levi, Primo. *Survival in Auschwitz* (New York: Simon & Schuster, 1996).

Levi, Primo. *The Periodic Table* (New York: Everyman's Library Contemporary Classics Series, 1995).

Lewis, C. S. *A Grief Observed* (San Francisco: HarperOne, 2015).

Lightman, Alan. *Searching for Stars on an Island in Maine* (New York: Vintage Books, 2019).

Schulman, Andrew. *Waking the Spirit, A Musician's Journey Healing Body, Mind, and Soul* (New York: Picador, 2016).

Shapiro, Dani. *Devotion: A Memoir* (New York: HarperPerennial, 2011).

Smith, Patti. *M Train* (New York: Bloomsbury, 2016).

Stone, Tobias. "History tells us what may happen next with Brexit & Trump," www.medium.com, July 23, 2016.

Tafreshi, Babak. *The World at Night: Spectacular Photographs of the Night Sky* (London: White Lion Publishing, 2019).

Tillich, Paul. *The Courage to Be* (New Haven: Yale Univ. Press, 2014).

Thoreau, Henry D. *Walden* (London: Dent, 1995).

Tolstoy, Leo. *A Confession* (New York: Penguin Books, 2008).

Wohlleben, Peter. *The Hidden Life of Trees* (Vancouver: Greystone Books, 2018).

Contemplative Prose and Poetry

Bishop, Elizabeth. *Elizabeth Bishop, the Complete Poems: 1927-1979* (New York: Farrar, Straus & Giroux, 1983).

Dickinson, Emily. *The Essential Emily Dickinson* (New York: Ecco, 2016).

Harding, Paul. *Tinkers* (New York: Bellevue Literary Press, 2009).

Hughes, Langston. *The Collected Poems of Langston Hughes* (New York: Vintage Classics, 1995).

Mitchell, Joni. *Joni Mitchell: The Complete Poems and Lyrics* (New York: Three Rivers Press, 1998).

Robinson, Marilynne. *Gilead* (New York: Farrar, Straus & Giroux, 2020).

Woolf, Virginia. *To the Lighthouse* (Boston: HMH Books, 1989).

Nearing End of Life

Callanan, Maggie, and Patricia Kelley. *Final Gifts: Understanding the Special Awareness, Needs, and Communications of the Dying* (New York: Simon & Schuster, 2012).

Danticat, Edwidge. *The Art of Death: Writing the Final Story* (Minneapolis: Graywolf Press, 2017).

Egan, Kerry. *On Living* (New York: Riverhead Books, 2017).

Gawande, Atul. *Being Mortal: Illness, Medicine, and What Matters in the End* (New York: Henry Holt and Company, 2014).

Miller, BJ, and Shoshana Berger. *A Beginner's Guide to the End: Practical Advice for Living Life and Facing Death* (New York: Simon & Schuster, 2020).

Parkes, Colin Murray. *The Price of Love: The Selected Works of Colin Murray Parkes* (Oxfordshire: Routledge, 2015).

Pearson, Patricia. *Opening Heaven's Door: What the Dying Are Trying to Say About Where They're Going* (New York: Atria Books, 2015).

Weller, Francis. *The Wild Edge of Sorrow: Rituals of Renewal and the Sacred Work of Grief* (Berkeley: North Atlantic Books, 2015).

Illness and Transplant

Blackwell, Courtney K., Amy J. Elliott, Jody Ganiban et al. "General Health and Life Satisfaction in Children With Chronic Illness," *Pediatrics*, January 2019.

Smith, Mallory. *Salt in My Soul: An Unfinished Life* (New York: Penguin Random House, 2019).

Weill, David, MD. *Exhale: Hope, Healing, and a Life in Transplant* (Brentwood, TN: Post Hill Press, 2021).

Consciousness

Crick, Francis. *The Astonishing Hypothesis: The Scientific Search for the Soul* (New York: Scribner, 1995).

Radin, Dean. *The Conscious Universe: The Scientific Truth of Psychic Phenomena* (San Francisco: HarperOne, 2009).

Sacks, Oliver. *The Mind's Eye* (New York: Vintage Books, 2011).

Steffen, Edith, and Adrian Coyle. "'I thought they should know . . . that daddy is not completely gone': A Case Study of Sense-of-Presence Experiences in Bereavement and Family Meaning-Making," *OMEGA Journal of Death and Dying*, January 2017.

Tarrant, Jeff. *Meditation Interventions to Rewire the Brain: Integrating Neuroscience Strategies for ADHD, Anxiety, Depression & PTSD* (Eau Claire, WI: PESI Publishing & Media, 2017).

Afterlife

Champlain, Sandra. *We Don't Die: A Skeptic's Discovery of Life After Death* (New York: Morgan James Publishing, 2013).

Jackson, Laura Lynne. *The Light Between Us* (New York: The Dial Press, 2016).

Kean, Leslie. *Surviving Death, A Journalist Investigates Evidence for an Afterlife* (New York: Crown, 2017).

Radin, Dean, PhD. *Real Magic: Ancient Wisdom, Modern Science and a Guide to the Secret Power of the Universe* (New York: Harmony, 2018).

Stevenson, Ian. *Children Who Remember Previous Lives: A Question of Reincarnation* (Jefferson, NC: McFarland, 2016).

Tadd, Ellen. *The Infinite View: A Guidebook for Life on Earth* (New York: TarcherPerigee, 2017).

Tucker, Jim B. *Life Before Life: A Scientific Investigation of Children's Memories of Previous Lives* (New York: St. Martin's Griffin, 2008).

Weiss, Brian. *Many Lives, Many Masters* (New York: Fireside, 1988).

Resources

Ananur Forma, astrologer: www.astrologywithananur.com

Center for Innovative Phage Applications and Therapeutics, UC San Diego School of Medicine: www.medschool.ucsd.edu/Pages/default.aspx

Center for Organ Recovery & Education: www.core.org

Cystic Fibrosis Foundation: www.cff.org

Forever Family Foundation: www.foreverfamilyfoundation.org

Karissa Eve Dorman, medium: www.karissaevemedium.com

Kristin Bredimus Spiritual Consultancy: www.kristinbredimus.com

Libby Barnett, Reiki Healing Connection: www.reikienergy.com

Mettle Health, palliative care consulting: www.mettlehealth.com

National Hospice and Palliative Care Organization: www.caringinfo.org

National Alliance for Caregiving: www.caregiving.org

Organ donation: www.organdonor.gov

Sirrý Berndsen, medium: www.spiritoflight.com

The Leo Project in Honor of Caitlin O'Hara: www.leoproject.org

The Tintero Foundation for Translation and the Literary Arts: www.tintero.org

What Matters Now: www.whatmattersnow.org

Windbridge Research Center: www.windbridge.org

ABOUT THE AUTHOR

MARYANNE O'HARA is the author of the novel *Cascade*, which was *The Boston Globe* Book Club's inaugural pick and a finalist for the Massachusetts Book Award, and a story collection that was a finalist for the Flannery O'Connor Award for Short Fiction. She is the former associate fiction editor of the literary journal *Ploughshares*, has taught creative writing at Emerson College and Clark University, and has had her writing published in literary journals and recognized by artist grants programs of the Massachusetts Cultural Council and the St. Botolph Club Foundation.

Little Matches is inspired by a blog that Maryanne kept while her daughter, Caitlin, was waiting for a lung transplant. Since Caitlin's passing, she has also been certified by the University of Vermont's Larner College of Medicine as an end-of-life doula, so that she may better speak to the state of end-of-life care in our culture. She lives in Massachusetts with her husband.

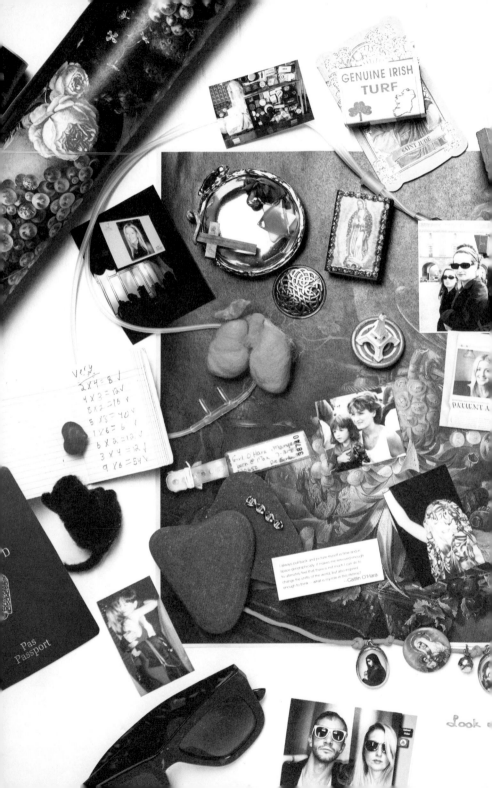